PERSONS NOT DISEASES

Persons Not Diseases

A Guide to Mind-Body-Spirit Medicine and Holistic Healing

JENNIFER BARRACLOUGH

Persons Not Diseases:
A Guide to Mind-Body-Spirit Medicine and Holistic Healing
Copyright © 2013 by Jennifer Barraclough

All rights reserved. Any use of the book without the author's consent is strictly prohibited.

ISBN-13: 978-1492196624
ISBN-10: 1492196622

Book design by Maureen Cutajar
www.gopublished.com

ACKNOWLEDGEMENTS

I would like to thank the clients, patients, colleagues and friends who have kindly written contributions for this book or given me permission to quote from their experiences.

CONTENTS

PART 1	Principles of Holistic Healing	11
PART 2	The Physical Level	21
PART 3	The Psychological Level	31
PART 4	The Spiritual Level	67
PART 5	Healing Relationships	89
PART 6	External Treatments	97
APPENDIX	Alphabetical list of complementary therapies	111
REFERENCES		113
ABOUT THE AUTHOR		117

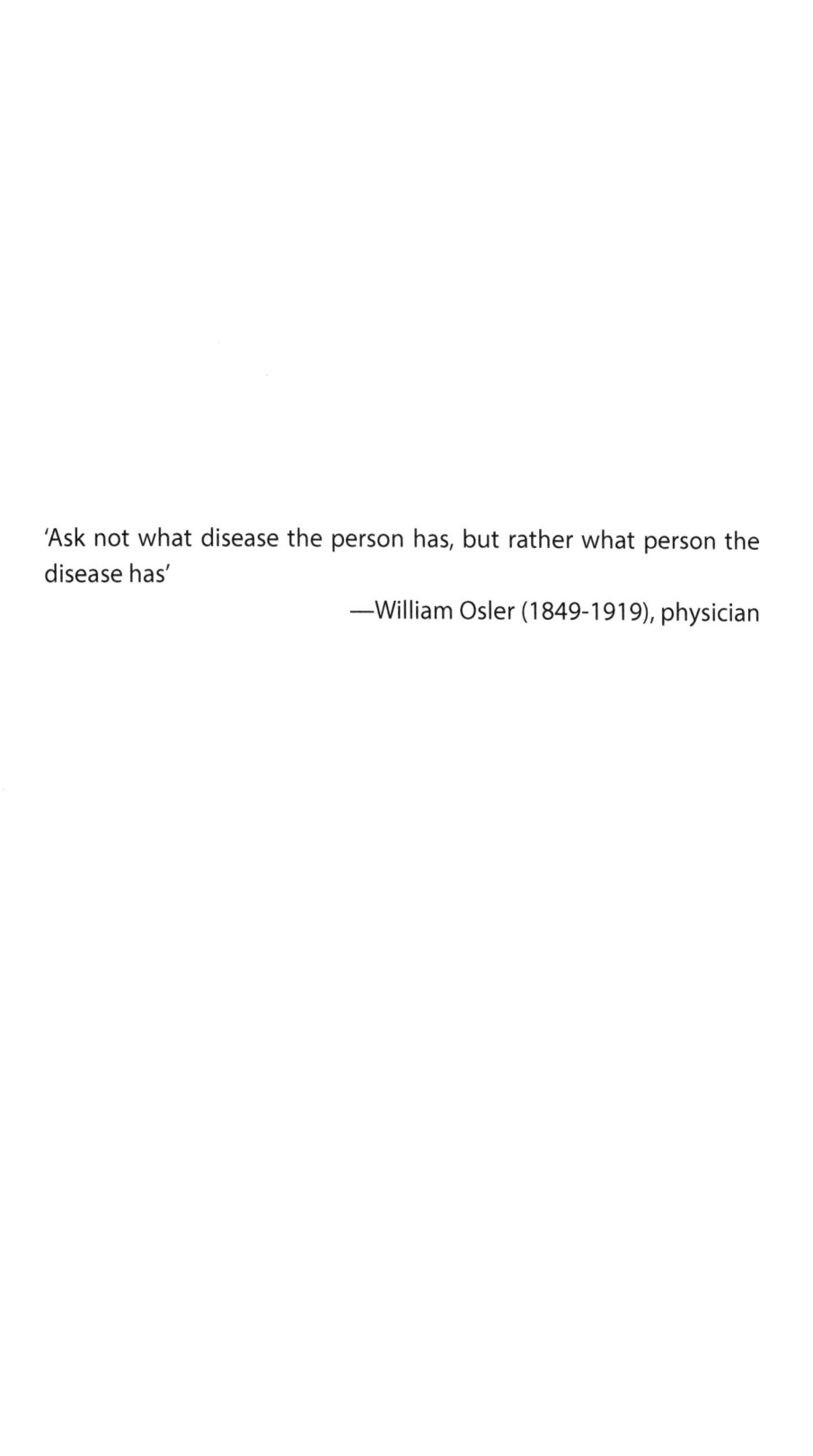

'Ask not what disease the person has, but rather what person the disease has'

—William Osler (1849-1919), physician

INTRODUCTION

Can I help my own recovery by improving my diet, taking more exercise, meditating, having a positive attitude, and reducing my stress levels? Can I use therapies like acupuncture, homoeopathy and herbal medicines as well as drugs and surgery, or even instead of them? Where can I find good information about approaches like these? And why did I get this illness – does it have some meaning and purpose in my life?

Such questions are of vital importance to many of those who are coping with health problems in themselves or in their families, and who want to play an active part in controlling the symptoms and improving the medical prognosis. But many doctors, nurses and other clinicians with an orthodox background feel uncomfortable with them, being unable or unwilling to provide their patients with helpful guidance about 'natural healing' and 'the holistic approach', and sometimes responding in negative ways when they hear these terms.

This book gives a broad overview of holistic healing, with an emphasis on self-help methods which can be used either on their own or alongside mainstream medicine and surgery. It is intended for anyone who is dealing with sickness from day to day, whether in their own personal lives or through their work. The style and content, combining practical guidance and clinical case examples with references to background theory and research, is designed to suit both general readers and healthcare professionals.

The information given here is, of course, general in nature and not a substitute for expert diagnosis and treatment, and I would advise anyone interested in self-healing and natural therapies to have a conventional medical assessment as well. The book is not intended to discredit orthodox medicine, or to discourage readers from using orthodox treatments in situations where these have proven value.

I followed the orthodox route myself for the first half of my career. I qualified as a doctor in 1970 and spent the next 30 years working in England in a variety of settings, eventually specialising in the psychological aspects of cancer care. For a long time, the only treatment options I knew much about were drugs, surgery and radiation. Under the influence of my senior colleagues I had developed rather dismissive views towards what in those days was often called 'fringe', or less politely 'quack', forms of medicine. My opinion began to change when I took a job in a hospice, and realised the potential benefits of 'extras' like acupuncture, aromatherapy, music and art. Certain patients, besides choosing to take part in such therapies, had made major changes in their attitudes and way of life since their diagnosis and I observed that some, though not all, of these were surviving much longer than predicted. I also became more aware of the spiritual aspects of life and death – topics which had fascinated me during my teenage years but become sidelined by my scientific training. A chain of synchronous events then led me to start studying, and experiencing, the world of holistic healing and natural therapy myself.

My life changed when I moved to Auckland with my New Zealand-born husband. Rather than register as a medical practitioner in my new country, I took some further training and embarked on a second career as a life coach and Bach flower remedy practitioner. Working part-time enabled me to pursue wider interests including writing, animals and music. And, as I and my family and friends have grown older and developed a few health problems ourselves, I have learned something first-hand of what it is like to be both a patient and a carer.

The holistic approach has brought a more positive and creative dimension to my own life, work and health but I do not consider it a panacea. Orthodox medicine and surgery often achieve excellent results, and are the best first line of approach for many conditions including for example heart attacks, broken bones, cataracts and certain types of cancer. However, the widespread popularity of complementary and alternative medicine (CAM) in the general population (Harris 2012) makes it clear that the orthodox approach does not meet every need. Perhaps there is a growing awareness that the technological advances in medical investigation and treatment, marvellous though they are, are tending to eclipse those basic principles of healing which are rooted in ancient wisdom and increasingly being validated by modern research. Many people are hoping for more individualised and 'whole-person' care, for treatments which seem safer and more natural, for better control of their symptoms, for recovery from a condition which has been pronounced 'incurable' by the medical authorities, for a deeper understanding of why they became ill, and for a sense of greater choice and control as regards their own health.

I believe that orthodox medicine (sometimes described as allopathic, mainstream or conventional) and CAM (which includes natural therapies and the 'mind-body-spirit' approach), each with their respective strengths and shortcomings, can work well together and that for the best results they need to be combined with the active participation of patients themselves. 'Patients' is not really the ideal word to use in this context because it implies the passive acceptance of medical treatment rather than the active pursuit of self-healing. But, for want of a better term, I shall continue to refer to 'patients' in this book except when 'clients' or 'users' or 'sick persons' is clearly more suitable. And, continuing on the theme of terminology, when I refer to 'clinicians' this includes doctors, nurses, radiographers, physiotherapists, occupational therapists, dieticians, dentists, optometrists and other orthodox healthcare professionals.

There is no universal formula for healing. A holistic approach can include many different components, and details of the 'illness journey' are different in every case. People new to the approach often feel somewhat overwhelmed and confused by the wide range of interventions to choose from, not knowing quite where to start. This book is intended to give a balanced introduction. As a short overview of a large field, it is concerned with general principles, and cannot provide details of specific diseases or treatments although some of them will be mentioned to illustrate particular points. Similarly, though a selection of academic citations is included, it would have been impossible to provide references to every statement in the text or a thorough review of the medical literature.

Part 1 gives an outline of holistic healing. Subsequent parts deal with body, mind and spirit topics, relationships with others, and the choice of professional treatments. The holistic healing approach cannot be reduced to a step-by-step programme to be followed in a particular order, and different readers will find some suggestions more relevant than others to their own situation. Many of the clinical examples relate to my own special interest of cancer care, but the same principles apply to other conditions besides cancer. Not all of the theories and therapies mentioned are ones which I would endorse personally, but they are included for completeness.

Persons not diseases started life as a new edition of my earlier text *Focus on healing*, but though some of the previous material has been retained it has been largely reorganised, updated and rewritten and so turned out quite a different book. There are new original case histories and the following one, written by 'Joanna' from New Zealand, illustrates many of the points which will be discussed later on. Joanna has shown me copies of her hospital notes, and the medical details which I have inserted in brackets are taken from these.

JOANNA'S STORY

I arrived home, after a day working in a school, to find a message on my phone asking me to contact the Breast Centre to discuss my recent mammogram. I knew at once, being prone to assume the worst in all situations, that I had breast cancer. Unfortunately it was the Friday night before a long weekend, which meant I had three days to wait before I could confirm my belief. To add to my stress, it was Breast Cancer Awareness Month and everywhere I went I was confronted with pink posters, women waving collection boxes, and magazine stories about women bravely battling breast cancer. It was a nightmare.

When I finally reported to the Breast Centre, a biopsy and scan confirmed that yes I did have cancer, and that the lump was already rather large, although because of its position it could not be felt even by the medical staff. I was enraged. I drove home in a fury and vented my anger in an empty house by screaming and shouting, not my usual behaviour. I eventually realised that I would have to deal with the situation and arranged to visit my GP. She clarified my options – surgery either publicly or privately. As a former medical librarian I had a great deal of respect for the public system, and we made an appointment for the following week.

Things went smoothly from then on. I began telling people about my situation as I had to cancel work and pull out of a committee I was on. I was booked for surgery a week after my first appointment and spent the time reading up on cancer, particularly Ian Gawler's book *You can conquer cancer*. Meditation and healthier eating took up my time and I began to feel more positive.

The operation (left mastectomy with axillary node dissection) went smoothly and I returned home after three days to be visited regularly by the district nurses who seemed impressed by the speed of my recovery. However, my growing confidence was shattered on my follow up appointment. I was told I had so many involved lymph nodes that I almost certainly had secondary cancer. (The breast tumour was an infiltrating lobular carcinoma, 60 mm in maximum dimension, grade 2, ER and PR positive. It had spread to 10 of the 12 lymph nodes examined). Again I was overcome with rage and thought of people in my life who I felt had caused this, a reaction which took some time to deal with.

Two scans and an MRI later it was confirmed that I had secondaries on my spine (the bone scan at this time was reported as showing metastatic lesions in the thoracic and lumbar vertebrae, and an MRI 'confirmed extensive metastatic disease'). At the time I did not understand the full significance of this – my main reaction was one of joy that I was not to be given chemotherapy or radiotherapy, since it was already too late to stop the cancer spreading. I had a lot to learn. (Joanna was prescribed hormonal therapy in the form of anastrozole, or Arimidex, an aromoatase-inhibiting drug which inhibits the synthesis of oestrogen, to 'give her some months of quality life'. She took it for five years.)

I had been told by a friend that the Cancer Society provided massages at subsidised rates, so I booked myself in at once. I met a marvellous woman who had had breast cancer herself and who became a very good friend. Through her I learned about a therapy called Body Talk, which I still receive on an occasional basis. I also enrolled in classes at the Society for yoga, relaxation and sleep improvement. I joined a group which met weekly for three months and learned meditation, healthy eating and positive thinking. Homework included watching funny DVDs. I attended two weekend courses for women with cancer, held at a health resort in the country. I went to Reiki, the Encore swimming programme, Pink Pilates, and a spiritual healer. I joined Sweet Louise, a new group for women with secondary breast cancer (www.sweetlouise.co.nz). All through this time I continued to feel fine, and always had clear blood tests, although it was a year before I learned that this was both unusual and significant. One oncologist told me that the cancer would get me in the end, despite my apparent healthy state.

After three years, the oncologists decided I should have another scan to see why I was still alive. Two weeks before Christmas, I was given the news that my original diagnosis must have been wrong and that I had never had secondaries. In fact I did discover that the white spots on my spine were still showing in the latest scan, though apparently of unknown origin. I was euphoric at this reprieve from an unhappy fate. I hugged the oncologist. I rang my family. I rang everyone who had helped me. I told the chemist. I told the woman in the wine shop where I bought champagne. I told the barista in my favourite café – I don't have cancer any more.

It is now seven years since I was first diagnosed with breast cancer, and four years since I was cleared of having secondaries. However I do not say I bravely battled breast cancer and won. I do not call myself a cancer survivor. I have spent too much time with women whose breast cancer killed them, despite their best efforts, to be complacent about my future immunity. I still maintain, as best I can, my 'healthy' routine. I no longer eat meat or dairy products. I practise meditation, somewhat erratically. I go to holistic cancer conferences and retreats when I can. I read cancer books when I find them.

I believe that a long period of stress in my work life led to a breakdown in my immune system which allowed some cells to 'behave badly'. I think this period also revived memories of some unhappy childhood interactions, although this insight came only recently. However I had managed to sort out the work problems, and am now resolving some other unhappy situations in my life. I believe I will need to work on my emotional issues as long as I live, as well as leading as healthy a life as possible to keep the cancer at bay.

I have strong feelings about the whole breast cancer industry, or at least the orthodox industry. I dislike the 'pink' image, and the amount of attention this form of cancer gets compared with other less 'glamorous' cancers. Where are the blue buses urging men to get their testicles checked, or the books with twenty personal accounts of 'my struggle with bowel cancer'? I also feel the present mainstream system of treatment is inadequate. When I said to one oncologist that it would be helpful to ask women about their life situations and stress levels, he said 'We only deal with medical things.' However it seems to me that cancer comes out of one's life, and a cancer diagnosis is a signal that there are issues which need attention. There are many good people, fortunately, who are working in the holistic area and help is available to those who are prepared to go looking.

* * *

Joanna was diagnosed with breast cancer in 2005 and at the time of writing in 2013 she remains well. It is not known whether the original diagnosis of bone secondaries was wrong, or whether her continued survival in good health is the result of her taking control of her condition through practical changes in lifestyle, the more open expression of emotions, and the use of complementary therapies.

In a letter which Joanna sent to the oncology clinic she expressed her appreciation for some aspects of the service, but suggested that patients could be offered fuller information about the medical aspects of their condition; fuller information about the support services available both within the hospital system and from outside agencies; that it would be helpful for staff to adopt a more positive and encouraging attitude; and that, rather than regarding the cancer as an 'isolated factor', recognise its relation to the patient's history and way of life.

PART 1

Principles of Holistic Healing

DEFINITIONS

The words 'holism' and 'healing' are both derived from the Greek *holos* meaning 'whole, all, entire, total' and it is often said that 'the whole is more than the sum of its parts'. Many of the tenets of the holistic approach are very old, dating back to the physicians of Ancient Greece, or to the healing systems of the East including Traditional Chinese Medicine and Ayurveda, but are still just as relevant today. Many of them sound simple and obvious but are often neglected in clinical practice. Many are fully compatible with the mainstream approach but some, being based on paradigms very different from Western science, are controversial.

The following definition comes from the website of the American Holistic Medical Association (www.holisticmedicine.org, accessed 2012):

'Holistic medicine is the art and science of healing that addresses care of the whole person – body, mind and spirit. The practice of holistic medicine integrates conventional and complementary therapies to promote optimal health, and prevent and treat disease by addressing contributing factors.

'In practice, this means that each person is seen as a unique individual, rather than an example of a particular disease. Disease is understood to be the result of physical, emotional, spiritual, social and environmental imbalance. Healing, therefore, takes place naturally when these aspects of life are brought into proper balance. The role of the practitioner is as guide, mentor and role model; the patient must do the work – changing lifestyle, beliefs and old habits in order to facilitate healing. All appropriate methods may be used, from medication to meditation.

'All appropriate methods' may be drawn from the fields of orthodox medicine, complementary and alternative medicine, or self-help.'

Using the image of a triangle to represent the relationships between these three approaches, orthodox medicine would be placed at the bottom left-hand corner because of its 'left-brain' characteristics: rational and logical, concerned with things that can be perceived through the five senses and preferably measured in numerical terms, governed by linear cause-and-effect.

At the bottom right-hand corner is complementary and alternative medicine with its more 'right-brain' nature: intuitive, creative, open to the intangible and metaphorical, focusing more on the big picture than fine detail of its separate parts.

These descriptions apply to the extremes of the two approaches, representing the yang (masculine) and yin (feminine) faces of healthcare. Neither of the extremes is sufficient on its own for healing, and neither of them is risk-free. There is a need for them both, and in practice they can overlap considerably. The line along the base of the triangle indicates that they are joined on a continuum and that there is scope for variation between them.

In prime position at the apex of the triangle is the person who contributes to his or her own healing through making changes in practical lifestyle and mental outlook, and through motivation to get well, and is connected with the other two points through a co-operative partnership with healthcare professionals.

The centre of the triangle is the integrative form of practice which comes from combining all three elements.

Some people who claim to be using the 'holistic approach' are just taking a dietary supplement or having regular massages, and though such single interventions can be helpful, the approach really includes much more than this and is about changing several aspects of life in ways which will be different in each case.

WHO CAN BENEFIT FROM HOLISTIC HEALING?

The holistic approach can be used for a wide variety of reasons and in many different settings.

Some users have serious life-threatening diseases, for example it is estimated that at least 50% of people with a recent diagnosis of cancer have tried one or more forms of CAM. Complementary therapies have been successfully introduced in some palliative care and oncology centres, as described in my earlier book *Enhancing cancer care*.

Other users are seeking help for the many chronic conditions such as diabetes, high blood pressure, coronary heart disease, arthritis, irritable bowel syndrome, neurological diseases and skin diseases which are prevalent in developed countries today. Western medicine cannot provide cures for most of these disorders and long-term medication, though bringing partial relief, often has unwanted effects.

A third group of users include people in reasonably good health who are looking for natural methods of treating minor ailments, enhancing their well-being, preventing disease, or reducing the impact of stress in their lives.

Many of the principles of the holistic approach are fully compatible with the orthodox one. Most holistic practitioners respect, and are willing to co-operate with, the world of orthodox medicine and while only a fanatic would claim that the approach is a valid alternative to the many effective medical and surgical interventions available today, it does mean that powerful drugs and technologies could be used more selectively, often being supplemented and sometimes being replaced by other means. There is however a certain amount of scepticism towards the field, and it sometimes provokes heated controversy.

TREATING THE PERSON NOT THE DISEASE

Two phrases often heard in holistic healing circles are 'treating the whole person' and 'treating the person, not the disease'.

Modern medicine is so complex that it has unavoidably become highly specialised, and undoubtedly this specialisation has led to many worthwhile advances in prevention and treatment which would not have been possible otherwise. Its downside is the fragmentation of care. It is not easy for different disciplines, often working in separate locations, to collaborate with each other even though it is known that there are links between apparently separate body systems and body parts, for example the association of gum disease with heart disease and with certain types of cancer. Links between body and mind, for example between mental depression and a long list of physical disorders, are especially likely to be missed in clinical practice.

The knowledge about anatomy, physiology and biochemistry which forms the foundation of orthodox medicine is hugely impressive in its complexity and scope. Yet, despite having so much detailed information to draw upon, the orthodox model still cannot offer a satisfactory explanation of how all the components of the living organism work together to form a functional whole. This miracle of co-ordination cannot be fully explained within the holistic model either, but holistic healers do emphasise that all aspects of the individual are interconnected and that the correct balance between them is essential for health. Physical disorders are often viewed as a manifestation of disharmony in the emotional, mental or spiritual spheres, or as responses to events in the person's life. To those with an allopathic training, some of the pathways described as mediating these connections may seem surprising, because they are often described in terms of energy systems rather than of anatomy, physiology and biochemistry.

The 'disease model' used in orthodox medicine has enabled great advances in the prevention and management of many conditions. Official classification systems set out criteria for diagnosing different diseases on the basis of various combinations of symptoms, signs and test results. Research studies carried out on groups of people with the same diagnosis yields knowledge about the causes, natural history and response to treatment of their disease.

If and when people who have suffered with 'medically unexplained symptoms' for some length of time are diagnosed as having a named disease, even one of quite a serious nature, they sometimes feel relieved about having their complaints explained and taken seriously, and knowing what they have to deal with.

But medicine is not an exact science, and the disease model has its limitations. Whereas some diseases are clearly defined by their characteristic pathology, others are not, and in practice many patients present to their doctors with one or more symptoms which do not fit with a recognised diagnosis. Diseases can be misdiagnosed, and significant ones can be missed, even after thorough medical assessment. Sometimes a serious condition is identified with confidence but the diagnosis is later called into question, as happened in Joanna's case described above. Physiological measurements such as blood sugar, blood pressure and body weight vary on a continuum, both between different people and at different times in the same person, and so numerical cut-off points between what is considered 'normal' or otherwise are somewhat arbitrary, and there will be many borderline cases. Another downside is that a set of negative assumptions and expectations can go along with diagnostic labels, and these can prove to be self-fulfilling.

There can be an important difference between feeling processed as a case of a certain disease, and feeling understood as a person having the experience of illness (Green, Carillo and Betancourt 2002). And, convenient though they are, terms like 'a diabetic' or 'an epileptic' carry the risk of defining people only in terms of what is wrong with them. Even if their orthodox medical management has been successful on a physical level, patients sometimes express dissatisfaction about being labelled as just another example of the condition in question, to be managed according to a set protocol, and feel that staff lack the knowledge or interest to look beyond their diseased part. By choosing to consult a holistic practitioner, they hope to feel valued as an individual with a unique psychology and life situation.

Diagnostic categories have only limited relevance to holistic healing. A good holistic treatment will be tailored to each person, in contrast to the 'one size fits all' approach of evidence-based medicine which is based on statistical analysis of large populations. A holistic practitioner will enquire about the presenting symptoms in some detail, but without necessarily assigning a diagnostic label, and without attempting to distinguish between categories such as 'physical or mental' and 'organic or functional' because all illness involves both body and mind. The risk of this approach is missing a disease condition which would be better treated by orthodox methods, which is a good reason for using holistic methods as complementary (alongside orthodox medicine) rather than alternative (instead of it).

When holistic healing is effective there will often be improvements in all aspects of health and well-being, as well as resolution of the target symptoms. But 'healing is not always curing'. In any case, cure is always an uncertain concept and reputable practitioners will never promise that a serious condition can be cured. This said, remarkable recoveries do happen occasionally, and some patients with advanced cancer and other serious diseases do experience prolonged survival or even cure. Often this follows some major shift in attitude or lifestyle, involving for example a dietary change, intensive meditation or the practice of forgiveness (Hirshberg and Barasch 1995; www.healingcancernaturally.com). However, sometimes the improvement just seems to happen by itself. Remarkable recovery, by definition, is a rare phenomenon and is unpredictable. Orthodox clinicians are often sceptical about reported cases, assuming that the original diagnosis was wrong, however many descriptions of 'spontaneous remission' from histologically proven malignancies can be found in the mainstream medical literature. Unfortunately, information about psychological aspects is often missing from these published accounts.

BALANCE

The term 'balance' has various applications relevant to the holistic healing approach. For example:

- Balance between body, mind and spirit,
- Balance between orthodox medicine, CAM, and self-help,
- Balance between the benefits and risks of different treatments,
- Balance between the conflicting information and advice to be found both in the academic literature and the general media,
- Balance between the perspectives of patients, relatives and clinicians.

Some enthusiasts lose their sense of balance by going to extremes which do more harm than good, for example following strict diets which lead to emaciation, nutritional deficiencies or eating disorders; taking excellent care of their physical bodies, but continuing to live with the stress caused by an unhappy marriage or work situation; meditating for many hours each day but not taking any exercise or brushing their teeth properly; spending their life savings on some new 'miracle therapy' which has not been properly tested; or becoming so obsessed with health-related issues that they neglect other domains of life relating to work and leisure, home and garden, finances, relationships with family and friends, and spirituality.

POSITIVE FOCUS

Whereas orthodox medicine is mainly focused on what is wrong with people, the holistic approach at its best is also concerned with what is 'right', with enhancing general well-being and encouraging the expression of individual interests, talents and values. A serious illness can bring out strengths of personality, enabling patients to realise what is really important to them and live more authentic lives, whether or not they experience physical improvement or recovery. Many natural therapies, such as aromatherapy and massage, are pleasant to receive and few of them carry much risk of distressing or dangerous side-effects.

Making the experience of illness and its treatment as pleasant and constructive as possible is obviously worthwhile for humane reasons and there is also substantial evidence that a 'positive' mindset tends to promote good health and recovery from illness, whereas a 'negative' one has the opposite effect.

THE CHALLENGES OF RESEARCH

Opponents of the holistic approach often claim that the benefits of unorthodox treatments are unproven. New therapeutic methods are not likely to be brought into state-funded healthcare systems unless there is published evidence to support their use.

Evaluating the holistic approach certainly presents real challenges. Some aspects of natural healing, being more aligned with philosophy and religion than with science, are impossible to assess with an experimental technique. Many holistic healers with flourishing practices 'know' that their methods work and are not interested in trying to prove this to a sceptical medical establishment. Many individual CAM therapies are in fact now well supported by published research, and there are several specialised journals devoted to the field as well as websites such as nccam.nih.gov and www.rccm.org.uk. However some of the evidence is conflicting and the methodology of some studies is open to criticism.

The 'gold standard' methodology used in orthodox medical research is the randomised controlled trial (RCT) in which the efficacy of the approach being tested, usually a new drug, is compared with that of a placebo. The whole process, from selection of patients to details of the treatment given, is standardised as far as possible. Trials are 'blinded' so that neither patients nor investigators are told whether they are receiving the placebo or the real drug. The RCT is suitable for evaluating some individual complementary therapies in some clinical situations though for some interventions, massage and aromatherapy for example, a valid 'sham' or placebo version is difficult or impossible to devise. The RCT is less appropriate when applied to the holistic approach in general, for reasons such as the following:

- CAM therapy regimes should be individualised. In homoeopathy, for example, different patients with the same condition might be prescribed any one of many different remedies, in different doses, depending on the precise nature of their complaints and on their personal characteristics, in keeping with the principle of treating the patient not the disease. This precept has often been ignored in clinical trials which give the same treatment to all participants,
- Several therapies are often used in combination. A truly holistic approach which addresses body, emotions, mind and spirit requires more than one kind of intervention. For maximum benefit, changes in lifestyle and mental attitude are required as well as compliance with the specific treatment under study,
- Patients' beliefs, attitudes, choices and motivation are important in the success or otherwise of the approach. Those with strong views for and against it will not co-operate with being randomised in a clinical trial,
- Outcomes may not be clear-cut. 'Healing is not always curing'; overall quality of life, and patient satisfaction, need to be considered as well as quantitative measures of symptom control or length of survival,
- Funding may be difficult to obtain, either because the therapies have little commercial application or because grant-giving bodies are prejudiced against them,
- CAM practitioners and academic medical researchers tend to work in different settings, so that opportunities for collaboration between them seldom arise in the natural course of events.

Therefore both the strengths and the limitations of the holistic approach may be better appreciated by using research designs other than the RCT. These include descriptive qualitative studies, and individual case histories. On a personal note, most of the published RCTs of Bach flower remedies have concluded that they are no better than placebo, but over 80% of the clients treated by myself and my colleagues in clinical practice have reported a positive response.

Good results for patients with cancer and other conditions are reported from centres such as Penny Brohn Cancer Care (formerly the Bristol Cancer Help Centre) in England, the Gawler Centre in Australia, and the Gerson Clinics in Mexico and Hungary. It must be remembered that those who attend the residential courses at such centres are self-selected people who are strongly committed to their own healing, and there would be insurmountable difficulties in carrying out randomised controlled trials.

Another aspect of evaluation involves the financial cost of treatment. Valid cost-benefit comparisons between the holistic and orthodox approaches are difficult or impossible to make. Self-help practices such as taking exercise or meditating, which have been shown to be helpful for both prevention and management of disease, cost nothing at all. CAM therapies in general are much cheaper than many medical and surgical procedures. The difference is that most orthodox treatments are available through state-funded healthcare systems, whereas the alternatives usually need to be paid for by users themselves.

PART 2

The Physical Level

This section will be relatively brief, because the main focus of this book is on psychological aspects, and there are numerous other books and websites which describe the physical aspects of sickness and healing in more detail and with more authority than I would be able to do.

In orthodox medical and surgical settings, both investigation and management are usually considered in physical terms alone. Although many cases of disease can apparently be successfully prevented or treated on this level, most holistic practitioners believe that the health of the body depends on the state of the mind and spirit, and that these must be addressed before true healing can occur. Material factors, though still important, need be considered in relation to other aspects of being. For example, people who neglect to take good care of their bodies – whether because of mental health problems, excessive involvement in work, or overindulgence in the pleasures of life – are likely to be more vulnerable to infections, toxins and other biological pathogens.

'To keep the body in good health is a duty, otherwise we shall not be able to keep our mind strong and clear' The Buddha

Measures such as eating a good diet and taking regular exercise can make significant contributions to both prevention and recovery for a whole range of disorders, and it is seldom too late to benefit from adopting a more healthy lifestyle. One of today's leading experts in this field is Dr Dean Ornish and the recommendations on his website www.ornishspectrum.com are based on scientific research and also emphasise the human qualities of pleasure, freedom, compassion and a sense of control.

The physical environment is also of great importance and in addition to avoiding dirt, damp, overcrowding and extremes of temperature, the holistic approach includes the 'green' ideals of respecting and living in harmony with nature. This would mean avoiding chemical or electromagnetic pollution, choosing fresh organic foods and pure water, and seeking for natural beauty in terms of sights, sounds and scents.

DIET AND NUTRITION

Diet and nutrition are very important in relation to maintaining health and recovering from illness. However there is a great deal of inconsistent advice about these subjects on offer from different sources. I do not claim to be an expert myself, but in this section I will aim to give an overview of current guidelines, and discuss some psychological aspects.

'Diet' refers to the type and quantity of food consumed, with its varying combination of proteins, fats, carbohydrates, fibre, vitamins, minerals and water. Some dietary components, after being broken down by digestive processes, are absorbed from the gut into the bloodstream as 'nutrition' for the body and brain, fuelling energy requirements and providing the materials needed for growth and repair. Other components, insoluble fibres for example, are not absorbed but are important for stimulating bowel activity and the elimination of waste. As discovered in recent years, diet also has a big influence on the make-up of the 'microbiome', the community of bacteria and other microorganisms which live in the body and help to determine its state of health.

Dietary factors make a large contribution to the development of the degenerative diseases which are so common in Westernised societies, as well as to the current obesity epidemic. Too much animal fat, sugars, fried foods, processed foods and drinks overload the body with toxins and excess calories, without providing enough key nutrients.

The pattern of eating and drinking, as well as the actual content of the diet, affects health and well-being. Going too long between meals, which includes missing breakfast, or failing to drink enough water can exacerbate headaches, constipation and many other symptoms. Sitting down at a dining table for a leisurely meal with family or friends is better than eating 'on the go' and in a rush.

Dietary measures are established as part of the management of many conditions including for example diabetes, renal disease, cardiovascular disease, liver disease, celiac disease and cases of allergy or intolerance to certain foods. How far the prognosis of other common major diseases can be improved by making changes in diet is not so easy to assess because patients' motivation, or lack of it, has such a big effect on compliance with randomised controlled trials. The Ornish studies indicated that a low-fat vegetarian diet has benefits for patients with prostate cancer. Surprisingly, studies looking at diet in relation to the prognosis of breast cancer have had mixed results although, looking at the overall evidence, it is probably wise for women who are concerned to prevent the development or recurrence of this disease to reduce their intake of animal fat, including dairy products, to eat plenty of vegetables and to avoid gaining excess weight, all of which is good advice for anyone. They may also wish to avoid alcohol, because though having one or two drinks per day helps to protect against heart disease, even a small amount of alcohol increases the risk of breast cancer.

Most experts recommend that everyone should limit their consumption of red meat, especially fatty meat, dairy produce, sugars, processed items, preservatives and additives. It is better to focus on fresh plant-based foods including a variety of vegetables, fruits, nuts, herbs and spices, with fish and poultry. One well-studied pattern of eating which has been shown to protect against cardiovascular disease (Estruch 2013) is the 'Mediterranean diet' characterised by a high intake of olive oil, fruit, nuts, vegetables and cereals; a moderate intake of fish and poultry; a low intake of dairy products, red meat, processed meats, and sweets; and wine in moderation, consumed with meals.

However, some of the other dietary systems which have become popular in recent years make rather different recommendations. For example various authorities advocate cutting out all fats, all sugars, or all grains and sources of gluten; some recommend eating plenty of animal protein, others recommend only plant-based foods. The Stone Age diet, the Wheat Belly diet, the Raw Food diet and the Blood Type diet are among the many systems which have become fashionable in recent years, along with a host of special weight-reduction diets including many which are ineffective and carry risks to health.

There is also a great deal of inconsistent dietary advice on with regard to individual substances such as soy, coffee, chocolate, wheat, salt, alcohol and even water. Perhaps such items could be good in small amounts but not in large ones, protect against some diseases while increasing the risk of others, or vary in their effects depending on the individual's genome (genetic make-up) and microbiome, and on the overall composition of the diet. Coffee, for example, helps to protect against several conditions including Alzheimer's, Parkinson's, diabetes, cirrhosis, gallstones, gout, some cancers, cardiovascular disease, stroke and mental depression. On the debit side it can exacerbate gastric ulcers, glaucoma, anxiety and insomnia; create dependency; and decrease the efficacy of homoeopathic remedies. On balance, although many natural therapists disapprove of it, drinking coffee appears to reduce all-cause mortality and to be good for health. However, its effects depend on the amount consumed, the method of preparation, whether milk or sugar is added, and on individual metabolism.

Personal beliefs and expectations about food can modify its effects on the body. The conviction that a certain food will trigger an allergic reaction or a headache may be self-fulfilling to some degree, as well as giving rise to a lot of worry. Someone who vomited on one occasion after a chicken dinner may become conditioned to be sick again if and when they eat chicken in future, even if the previous incident should have been a 'one-off' due to that particular portion of chicken being infected, or even because the vomiting was due to some cause quite unconnected with the meal. Conversely, people can put exaggerated faith in certain items of diet, believing that they will get better if they eat enough berries or asparagus or whatever the latest 'superfood' is said to be.

The benefit of taking vitamin and mineral supplements is also uncertain. Some of these can certainly be harmful in excess. Other debated topics include the value of organic foods, of raw foods, of detox regimes, and the safety of GM crops and of microwave cooking.

Some alternative and complementary practitioners place great importance on dietary treatments. One of the best-known, long-established and also most demanding systems is that developed by Dr Max Gerson (www.gerson.org). There are no controlled trials, but many case reports of excellent results in cases of cancer and other conditions. A vivid personal account of receiving Gerson therapy for the treatment of melanoma can be found in the book *A Time to Heal* by my friend and colleague Beata Bishop.

It is likely that, for those few people who have the determination and will-power to follow demanding therapies such as this, belief in their value contributes to their benefits. This would help to explain the positive results which are claimed for various special diets which are quite different from each other.

Major dietary changes are not without risk. Certain regimes are deficient in essential nutrients, for example a vegan diet always needs to be supplemented with vitamin B12. The psychological aspects of eating and drinking are also important, because for most people food is among the major pleasures of life. Making major changes to established eating habits proves too much of a challenge for some to maintain, whereas others take it so seriously that they become obsessive and lose too much weight or develop eating disorders. Many special diets are expensive and time-consuming, and though they may be easy to follow when provided for groups attending a residential retreat, they can be incompatible with ordinary family and social life especially when other household members are not sympathetic or when there are few 'healthy' items on restaurant menus. They are even more difficult for those whose food choices are already limited by symptoms such as nausea or problems with swallowing. Some people are quite understandably more concerned with enjoying the present than with gaining possible long-term benefits, and are so unwilling to replace their favourite foods with ones they do not like. This is especially true if the illness fails to recover despite the special diet. Quotes from patients include 'If I've only got six months to live I don't want to spend it drinking green tea' and 'If I have another heart attack, and I survive it, I'm going to give up this diet and eat whatever I please.'

Perhaps the best advice can be summed up in such old sayings as 'everything in moderation' and 'a little of what you fancy does you good'. It is also true that also 'one man's meat is another man's poison' for there are both genetic and acquired variations in the way that different people respond to different foods. The body can withstand a good deal, and it is obvious that some robust individuals can get away without observing the dietary guidelines, for example Her Majesty Queen Elizabeth the Queen Mother apparently freely indulged her love of rich food and had a daily alcohol intake many times higher than the recommended limit, yet lived to be over 100.

To summarise the guidance in this section, it is best for most people to enjoy a good selection of fresh unprocessed foods in moderate amounts without getting too worried by the occasional lapse from 'healthy eating' guidelines, but some individuals do have special needs and will benefit from consulting a qualified dietician.

Interest in diet and health may extend to wider issues such as the welfare of farm animals and the conservation of the earth's resources. And there is some evidence that dietary improvements are more effective when combined with lifestyle changes such as taking more exercise.

EXERCISE

Taking regular exercise protects against many disorders including cardiovascular disease, diabetes, obesity, various cancers, osteoporosis, Alzheimer's, the common cold, and mental depression. It improves the strength of bones and muscles, oxygenation of the tissues, competence of the immune system, and mental well-being. But physical inactivity is endemic in the developed world, and has been identified as a major threat to health, maybe just as bad as smoking cigarettes. It often goes along with sitting down for long periods, which is harmful in its own right.

Like most things, exercise is best taken in moderation. Exercising too much can lead to musculoskeletal problems, hormone imbalance, damage to the heart and the risk of injury. Formerly inactive people just starting an exercise programme are best advised to work up gradually.

There are numerous ways to take exercise: everyday activities such as gardening, housework, going shopping on foot; all kinds of sport, swimming, dancing; special techniques such as yoga or tai chi. Even for people who are sick or disabled, some form of exercise such as passive movement underwater may be appropriate under the guidance of a physiotherapist.

Interestingly, it has been shown that taking exercise in the imagination produces some of the same physiological changes as the real thing.

One of the best and most natural ways to take exercise is simply walking outdoors, and this has the added benefits of exposure to sunlight and contact with the earth.

SUNLIGHT

Among the simplest, cheapest and perhaps most important ways of maintaining and improving health is getting some regular exposure to sunlight. Many people today are cut off from its benefits because they spend most of their time inside buildings or cars and, if they do go outside, cover their entire skin surface with clothing or sunscreen.

Moderation is important here. Health education programmes have focused strongly on the danger of developing skin cancer from exposure to the sun, and it is certainly true that too much of this can be damaging and that sunburn is always a bad thing. Too little sunlight, however, can result in vitamin D deficiency and an increased risk of many disorders including osteoporosis, multiple sclerosis, certain cancers and mental depression. Also, the safety of the chemicals in sunscreen creams has been questioned.

EARTHING

Whereas sunlight is only beneficial in moderate amounts, contact with the earth's energies is perfectly safe and preliminary studies indicate that 'earthing' or 'grounding' can improve health in numerous ways (Ober, Sinatra and Zucker 2010). This is thought to be because absorption of electrons from the earth into the body neutralises free radicals and so reduces the chronic inflammation which contributes to many forms of degenerative disease. People who seldom go out walking, wear shoes with insulating soles, or live and work in high-rise buildings are deprived of these benefits. Barefoot contact with grass or sand for at least half an hour per day is the most natural method of earthing but this is not always feasible, and through the use of special sheets and mats it is possible to be earthed while sleeping, working at a desk or driving a car.

SLEEP

The purpose of sleep is repair of the physical body and clearing of the mind. Lack of sleep, as everyone knows, impairs energy and general well-being. It disrupts endocrine and immune function, and is a risk factor for many medical conditions including cardiovascular disease, diabetes and obesity. Most adults need around seven hours sleep per night, though individual requirements vary, and the quality as well as the duration of sleep is important.

Many sick people suffer from disturbed sleep because of physical problems such as pain, mental problems such as worry, and the unwanted effects of drugs such as steroids and beta blockers. In hospitals, especially in intensive care units, sleep is frequently interrupted by noise or scheduled procedures. Even those in 'rest homes' often get woken up far too early in the morning. Lack of sleep is often a problem for carers, as well as for sick people themselves, and sometimes partners may do best to have separate beds or separate bedrooms to prevent one or both becoming sleep-deprived.

In certain circumstances the best option is to take sleeping pills, but while these can be useful on occasions, many people are rightly reluctant to take them every night. More natural aids to a good night's sleep include the following:

- Establishing a routine, so that you go usually to bed and wake up around the same time,
- Having a relaxing bed-time ritual such as a warm bath or reading,
- Avoiding eating or drinking too much late in the evening, but not going to bed hungry either. Sleep-promoting foods such as almonds, bananas, milk, oatmeal and wholewheat bread can be included in the last meal of the day,
- Avoiding excess tea, coffee and alcohol at any time,
- Avoiding heavy exercise in the evening,
- Avoiding bright lights, television and computer screens late in the evening,
- A comfortable bed, warm but not too hot,
- Curtains thick enough to keep out early morning light,
- Protection from noise and other disturbances as far as possible,
- Practising a calming affirmation, visualisation or relaxation technique when lying down to sleep.

AVOIDING POLLUTION

Many kinds of environmental pollutants, mostly man-made, are present in the air, water, soil and buildings of today. Chemical varieties include diesel fumes, industrial compounds, food additives, pesticides, artificial fabrics and dyes in clothing. Electromagnetic radiation in the atmosphere, due for example to computers, mobile phones, motors and power lines, has increased enormously in recent years and is no less real because it cannot be seen, heard or felt. Another form of pollution is noise, for example from road traffic, aircraft, construction and garden machinery. Many of these hazards have been shown to contribute to cancer, lung disease, heart disease, autoimmune disorders and other conditions.

Improving the safety of the environment requires action from governments and public health agencies. Ways in which individuals can protect themselves include eating fresh organic foods and rather than processed or tinned items, avoiding food and beverages from plastic containers especially if they have been microwaved, drinking filtered water, avoiding chemicals in the house or garden, wearing natural fibres, avoiding smoke and traffic fumes, reducing mobile phone and computer use, and favouring natural rather than artificial light.

APPRECIATING THE BODY

Many people fail to appreciate their bodies. Influenced by the latest trends in fashion and beauty, they criticise aspects of their appearance such as shape, size and colouring. They take for granted the wonderful complexity of all the continuous subconscious processes which sustain life, unless and until something goes wrong. They may dwell on health-related anxieties, perhaps worrying about developing a disease which runs in their family, or expecting to deteriorate after a certain age. Whether or not such negative attitudes actually contribute to causation of illness, they certainly cannot promote happiness or health. Louise Hay, one of the foremost self-help writers of modern times, continually advises 'loving your body' as a prerequisite to healing.

PART 3

The Psychological Level

This, the longest section of the book, presents some practical techniques and background theory from the complex field of mind-body medicine. More detailed coverage of these topics can be found in Dr Lissa Rankin's book *Mind over medicine*.

SELF-RESPONSIBILITY

While most conventional treatments place patients in a passive role, the holistic approach requires them to be proactive, making changes both in practical lifestyle and in attitudes of mind.

Sayings such as 'All healing is self-healing' and 'All healing comes from within' express the truth that although some form of external treatment may be needed, this can only succeed if the body's own recovery processes play their part. The repair of a surgical wound is an example. Many of the cures which are credited to drugs, surgery or CAM would probably have occurred on their own. The body has amazing self-healing powers, although these can be blocked by many different factors ranging from poor nutrition to negative beliefs.

There is some evidence that having a strong sense of autonomy is good for health, for example people whose jobs allow them little choice and control have a higher risk of coronary heart disease than those who feel empowered in their work environment (Bosma et al 1997). Patient participation in treatment decisions is widely believed to be associated with improved medical outcomes for various disease conditions. Clinicians can encourage autonomy by relating to their patients as equals rather than adopting an authoritarian stance, aiming for a co-operative partnership, and by making information readily available. They will find fewer of them seem difficult, dependent or demanding, and that they themselves do not feel so burdened by responsibility for their well-being. There are of course some patients who are not physically or mentally capable of making choices for themselves, some whose personality or cultural background inclines them to leave everything to the experts or to fate, and others who are disinclined to devote time and energy to their own healing and would rather just take some pills.

Though concepts of 'taking control of your own health' and 'self-responsibility' are so important in holistic healing, they are often misunderstood. Self-responsibility does not mean rejecting the benefits of professional treatment, or trying to cope alone without the love and support of others. Nor is it about 'blaming the victim' and making people feel that getting sick or failing to recover is their own fault. What it does mean is being well-informed, taking active steps towards good self-care, and participating in decisions about the management of illness.

Though some say that we 'create' all our own health problems, it seems to me that many aspects of illness are beyond personal control, especially in cases affecting children. Individuals cannot be held consciously responsible for having a genetic defect, being exposed to invisible environmental toxins, or developing a disease of unknown cause. Nobody should be made to feel 'I must have dome something wrong to attract this illness' or 'my cancer came back because I wasn't positive enough'.

If, after taking all reasonable keys towards healing, recovery has still not taken place there is no point in feeling guilty. It is more helpful to take a position of acceptance and surrender. This is not the same thing as hopelessly giving up, but means acknowledging that the situation cannot be changed at present; that it has perhaps developed for a reason and will eventually work out for good in the bigger scheme of things; and endeavouring to adapt to it in the best possible way.

SEEKING INFORMATION ABOUT CAUSES AND TREATMENTS

Today's media are full of information about health and healing. Looking up any common medical condition on Google will yield literally millions of hits. Medically themed documentaries and fiction are popular in magazines, newspapers, radio and TV. In many ways it is wonderful to have such an abundance of material freely available, but for lay people with a health problem the sheer volume of advice, some of it inconsistent, can seem quite overwhelming. Those with sensitive personalities may become fearful and hypochondriacal in reaction to continual reminders of what can go wrong with them.

It is difficult even for top medical experts to keep up to date with developments relevant to their own specialties, let alone with advances in other fields. Knowledge is always being updated, and some of the 'facts' which I learned at medical school would now be considered only partially correct or even completely wrong. New treatments are continually being introduced, and heralded as being more effective and safer than the old ones, though not all these claims will stand the test of time.

Despite the abundance of information, many aspects of health and sickness remain a mystery. Some people develop serious disease when they are still young, in the absence of any known risk factors and despite having looked after themselves well, and apparently leading a happy well balanced emotional life even if it could be surmised that they harbour conflicts and negative beliefs in their unconscious minds. Others live to a ripe old age although they have abused their bodies in various ways or gone through major psychological traumas. Similarly, it is often impossible to explain why the prognosis of the same condition can vary so much between different cases, with some proving fatal and others going on to complete recovery.

It would be nice to be able to identify a single cause for any given illness, and to know that recovery would follow when that cause was removed. Many popular self-help books dealing with selected aspects of health give the impression that the vast majority of human ills are due to a single factor, whether this is eating the wrong food or being unable to process emotional trauma from the past. But in reality, things are seldom so simple. Much disease is the end result of a combination of many different factors – genetic and environmental, physical and psychological, often going back for many years. To take the example of a heart attack, the obvious immediate cause is usually a blockage of one of the coronary arteries, and with modern treatment the circulation can often be successfully restored. But the condition may well recur if the patient has a heavy loading of underlying risk factors. Some of these can be tackled by changes in lifestyle: improving the diet, taking more exercise, losing excess weight, stopping smoking, reducing excess drinking, modifying negative mental attitudes and better management of stress. Others such as a strong family history, a low birth weight, experience of adversity in childhood or even in the womb, and some would say the destiny of the soul, cannot be changed.

Even if one main cause can be identified and dealt with, other treatment measures may be needed to reverse or halt the progress of the disease. For smoking-related conditions, for example, giving up smoking is an essential part of management but is seldom sufficient on its own.

Considering all these complexities and uncertainties, how much can the power of the mind really influence physical health?

MIND OVER MATTER: CLINICAL EVIDENCE

The power of the mind to shape material reality has been repeatedly stated down the ages by spiritual teachers and self-help experts, for example 'What we think, we become' (The Buddha) and 'Your life is a mirror of your consistent thought' (Napoleon Hill).

What exactly is meant by the 'mind' is a question which has long been debated. The conventional view in neurology and psychiatry is to regard the mind as a product of brain activity, but alternative theories propose that the brain is only 'a tool of the mind', interpreting its signals like a radio set tuned to receive certain frequencies, that the mind pervades the heart, gut and other organs besides the brain, and also extends outside the individual body to merge with other minds and with the 'universal mind' over time and space. The mind is not a 'thing' which can be localised anatomically or analysed chemically. It can be better understood as a process, concerned with the flow of energy and information, only a small part of which is present in conscious awareness at any one time. To use a more modern analogy, perhaps data is mainly stored in the 'cloud' of the mind rather than just in the 'computer' of the brain.

The mind-body connection has been extensively researched in recent decades but there is still much more to be learned. This connection works both ways, and the links between psychological factors and physical health are complex ones. 'Psychological factors' include emotions, thoughts, attitudes, beliefs, intentions and expectations. These are closely intertwined and although they sometimes need separate consideration, I will sometimes use the general term 'mindset' to cover them all.

Perhaps the most widely known and accepted piece of evidence that the mind can influence physical health comes from the placebo effect and its opposite, the nocebo effect. Analysis of placebo-controlled clinical trials leaves no doubt that the beliefs and expectations of patients themselves, and also of the clinicians who are treating them, contribute significantly to both the therapeutic and unwanted effects of many prescribed drugs. This is most strongly illustrated with psychotropics and analgesics. A similar phenomenon applies for certain surgical operations. There is of course a limit to this effect. Some people are more suggestible than others and there are some interventions, such as general anaesthetics, which are so powerful biologically that they work whether the patient believes in them or not.

Thoughts and expectations about illness, ranging from feeling ill after eating a certain food to dying at the same age as a parent did, certainly cause a lot of worry and may sometimes influence physiology so strongly that they become self-fulfilling prophecies. In one study, men who believed themselves to be at high risk of heart disease or stroke were indeed more likely to develop these conditions than those who believed they were at low risk, after allowing for physical factors (Gramling, Klein and Eaton 2008). Patients are sometimes observed to go into a rapid decline after being informed that there is something seriously wrong with them, even if they had few symptoms beforehand and the diagnosis was only made as a chance finding or as a result of a screening test. When I worked in a hospice I did not see any cases of the remarkable recovery from 'terminal' illness which are sometimes reported in other settings; could this be because of the pervading belief among patients and staff that all those receiving hospice care are destined to die quite soon? Clinicians can unwittingly reinforce negative expectations by telling patients that their condition is incurable, or is bound to get worse with increasing age. Conversely, an encouraging prognosis from a medical authority or a session with a charismatic healer will tend to promote recovery. I am not advocating that a serious diagnosis or prognosis should be withheld from patients who want to understand their situation and arrange their lives accordingly, but it is important to keep open-minded about the future and not to destroy hope.

Holistic healers have long believed that most disease is rooted in psychological imbalance. The idea that psychological factors can contribute to physical illness, by increasing vulnerability to material pathogens, is now being taken seriously in orthodox circles too. To examine the question of whether psychological make-up can affect health status in later years, several long-term follow-ups have been conducted on large groups of people who appeared to be free of disease at the beginning of the study. It has been found that the long-term persistence of negative moods, expectations, attitudes and beliefs predisposes towards various kinds of ill-health, including major organic conditions such as heart disease and cancer. For example, follow-up of people who have suffered from clinical depression reveals greatly increased morbidity and mortality, and depression is a well-established risk factor for heart disease (Bunker et al 2003). Even quite minor degrees of psychological imbalance, if sustained over time, may prove damaging (Russ 2012). It may also be that the apparent absence of negative emotions, due to deliberate suppression or unconscious repression, is especially harmful although this is obviously rather difficult to study.

Conversely, several researchers have reported that people whose attitudes and emotions are predominantly positive enjoy longer and healthier lives than those with a habitually negative outlook (Chida and Steptoe 2008). The findings are not entirely consistent; one study found that optimists tend to live longer than pessimists (Giltay, Geleljnse and Zitman 2004) and another found the reverse (Lang, Weiss and Gerstorf 2013).

It may be that specific personality traits or types of psychological conflict predispose to specific medical conditions, for example many though not all studies conclude that chronic hostility, anger and impatience are risk factors for cardiovascular disease. The concept of a 'cancer-prone personality', marked by the tendency to comply with others' expectations, suppress any negative feelings and maintain a polite social manner, is even less well supported by research although my own clinical experience has inclined me to believe it contains some truth. Other maladaptive traits which have been implicated as contributing to illness of various kinds include intolerant and critical attitudes, an exaggerated need for control, and feeling over-responsible for others. These reported associations refer to general trends which do not apply in every case; many different factors contribute to disease and there is certainly no hard-and-fast correlation between particular mental attitudes and particular conditions.

Another group of studies has examined the question of whether a person's attitude towards a disease which has already been diagnosed has an effect on the medical outcome. Not surprisingly, it has consistently been found that a 'helpless-hopeless' mindset tends to predict a poor prognosis. Other attitudes which tend to hinder both psychological adjustment and physical self-healing include self-blame, self-pity, anger, resentment, and passive resignation.

The more constructive attitudes tend to be those which involve a proactive stance, with a sense of hope and of having some control over the future. Those who perceive their illness as a challenge and approach it with a 'fighting spirit' attitude are often admired though it is possible to take this too far, leading to obsessive preoccupation with disease-related topics, or to exhaustion from intensive therapy regimes and drastic lifestyle changes. Some degree of 'denial' can be preferable, if this means not dwelling too much on the seriousness of the condition, and focusing attention on pleasanter aspects of life.

Moods and attitudes are not always fixed over time, nor can they be easily disentangled from physical state or behavioural factors. Everyone has to find his or her own best way of adjusting to illness, and it is unwise to make value judgements by labelling coping styles as 'good' or 'bad', 'right' or 'wrong'.

Beliefs and attitudes towards an illness often reflect longstanding beliefs and attitudes of a general nature, relating for example to the presence or absence of self-worth, whether the world is perceived as a benevolent or a hostile place, whether life seems an exciting journey or a continual struggle. They may have been instilled from early childhood, as part of the culture of the family or society, or have been imprinted by some critical experience in adult life. They are often taken for granted, perhaps not even consciously recognised, but can be likened to continuously running mental programmes exerting powerful effects on the worldview and behaviour of the person concerned. Even if they are challenged, and seen to be damaging and illogical, they are not easy to release. Special techniques, some of which are listed in the Appendix, exist for identifying, and changing, 'maladaptive' states of mind.

MIND OVER MATTER: POSSIBLE MECHANISMS

How are mind-body influences actually mediated? There appear to be several possible mechanisms, some of them grounded in mainstream biological disciplines such as psychoneuroimmunology (PNI), epigenetics and neuroscience, and others coming from the more controversial field of energy medicine. Broadly speaking, a positive mindset promotes relaxation and boosting of the body's immune defences, and a negative mindset promotes the stress response which renders the body more vulnerable to disease. In addition there are often behavioural factors involved, for example increased smoking, drinking or risk-taking by those who feel unhappy or stressed.

Emotional state affects the mix of hormones and cytokines which is continuously being released into the bloodstream and influences all aspects of physiology. The classic example is the 'fight-or-flight response' or 'stress response' in which there is activation of the sympathetic nervous system with increased secretion of chemicals including adrenaline, noradrenaline and cortisol, leading to increases in heart rate and blood pressure and numerous other changes. In the short term these may be helpful for dealing with a crisis, but if sustained over long periods they are detrimental to health.

It was once believed that, once a person reached adult life, the development of their brain came to a halt and any subsequent changes could only involve deterioration. This has now been shown to be untrue. The term 'neuroplasticity' refers to the ability of the brain to change, even in old age, in response to experiences, activities and predominant patterns of thought. Initially the changes are chemical ones, involving the balance of neurotransmitter substances being secreted. Eventually there are structural changes involving the pathways of connection between brain cells (neurones), the death of some brain cells and the production of new ones (neurogenesis). Many examples have been identified, relating for example to practising a skill such as playing a musical instrument, learning a new language, or meditating regularly; being exposed to a major psychological trauma such as warfare or an accident; or developing a substance addiction. Details can be found in Norman Doidge's book *The brain that changes itself*. It is exciting and empowering to realise that we may be able to change the 'hard-wiring' of our brains by changing our thoughts and behaviours, even if such change often requires sustained practice and motivation over time. However some acquired brain pathways are permanent, which could explain why people who have become physically dependent on alcohol can suddenly relapse after many years of total abstinence if they take just one single drink.

Changes in the body and brain, such as those summarised above, are mediated through variation in the expression of the genes. The basic composition of an individual's unique inborn genetic blueprint (genome), made up of sequences of DNA within the nucleus of each cell of the body, always remains the same. A small minority of individuals are born with a severe genetic disorder which will produce ill-effects no matter how favourable the environment. But the majority of people have a reasonably adequate set of genes and, though they may have a genetic vulnerability to certain diseases, whether they actually develop these or not depends to a large extent on which of their genes are switched 'on' or 'off' at different times of life. This in turn depends on what signals are being picked up by the receptors on the cell membrane. Some of these signals are chemical ones circulating in the bloodstream, including both the products of substances ingested, inhaled or absorbed from external sources, and the internally-generated hormones and cytokines mentioned above. Other signals are probably energetic rather than chemical. All of them, at least where responsible adults are concerned, are psychologically mediated to some degree because they depend on individual behaviours and perceptions, ranging from the choice of foods to the way of reacting to the challenges of life. A popular book on this subject is Bruce Lipton's *The biology of belief*.

Other theories of how mind-body effects are mediated include the concept of 'cellular memory', whereby the record of a person's past feelings and life experiences is stored not just in the brain but in other organs too. If this material includes repressed negative emotions, it can eventually give rise to physical pathology. Massage therapists describe the recall of mental traumas when certain parts of the body are being worked upon; there are many stories of transplant recipients taking on the personality characteristics of their organ donors. How these things could happen is not known, but it has been suggested that they involve the neuropeptides which are associated with different emotional states, or data in the energy fields which permeate the physical body.

The complexity of this field is illustrated by the following case history, in which the development of multiple physical symptoms can best be explained by the combination of unresolved emotional traumas and exposure to environmental toxins.

TERESA'S STORY

When I was 28 years old my husband and brother-in-law were killed by a drunk driver. The following evening I received a phone call from my boss and it was made clear that I had to return to work after the funeral and 'not to turn this into the worst thing that has ever happened to you'. I was completely traumatized and couldn't even walk into another room on my own without my mother coming with me, let alone think about going to work.

It was a high profile accident and I went to stay with my parents who kept the TV and radio switched off and the newspapers hidden from view. The police gave me a few sketchy details but I had many unanswered questions. Was my husband conscious? How exactly did he die? Did he suffer? The torment went on and on and I couldn't sleep for several nights even though I was medicated. The pain and anguish was horrific.

I returned to work after the funeral, that's how things were in 1978. There was no such thing as bereavement leave. In the company I worked for there was clearly no compassion either. I just simply had 'to get on with it' even though I was in no fit state to be working. It was a very surreal environment and the staff had been told not to talk to me about what had happened. Years later I discovered that it was considered the best way for me to 'get over it'.

Through a strange twist of fate, I had three appointments with a grief therapist who helped me enormously and I remember to this day the most important question she asked me 'How long do you want to be like this for?' I heard myself answer 'I want to be over it in a year'. Little did I know what was to come twelve years later, but at the time the question gave me a sense of taking some control over the sickening feelings of despair, horror and anguish. I was so low I prayed to God to take me in the night and was disappointed each morning to wake up and have to face another day.

As time went by, I began to feel better and by the end of the 12 months I had progressed enormously. However, there was more to come because during that year my mother was diagnosed with terminal cancer and passed away two years later, then eleven months later my father also passed away from cancer. Again I had to keep my, at times overwhelming, grief in check and keep working as I had quit my job and gone to work for myself. I had commitments to keep and staff to pay. Again, I simply had to 'get on with it'.

Slowly life took on normalcy again and eight years after the death of my husband I remarried and moved to another city where I knew just two people. It was not a welcome move but my new husband was transferred in his role so I had to leave behind what was left of my family, friends and support network I'd known all my life and who'd helped me through the trauma of the past few years.

The following year I began to get all manner of health problems from benign breast lumps, appendicitis, a hormonal imbalance and a host of unexplained aches, pains and symptoms. I saw nine specialist physicians in five years, was tested for neurological disorders including epilepsy and incorrectly diagnosed with multiple sclerosis, a tumour on an ovary and a premature aging condition. Some specialists simply said that there was something definitely wrong but they didn't know what. I respected their honesty but it didn't help me get better.

At about that time I was also exposed to pesticides in my workplace and not much was then known about chemical poisoning. My symptoms were severe and included chronic fatigue, sleepiness, confusion, anxiety, nausea, dyslexia, weight gain, headaches, distorted hearing, vision problems, fluid retention, painful joints, aching limbs, bowel problems, I felt cold and had multiple allergies. In my search for someone who could help me I saw one doctor who thought I might be suffering from unresolved grief. 'How ridiculous,' I thought. I had coped very well, hadn't I? I had got on with my life, hadn't I? I had a new marriage and a whole new life had opened up for me. How wrong I was!

Over the five years despite the many tests I became sicker and sicker and eventually had to resign from my management role as I had become incapable of working. I had become so confused that I couldn't find my way to work so my secretary drove to my home each morning so I could follow her car. I was eventually treated by an acupuncturist who asked me what had happened 12 years earlier. I answered that that had been when my husband was killed. He told me that I was like an engine running on one cylinder and that was how I felt. After a few treatments, he asked me if I felt like I'd been poisoned which was very interesting because I had been thinking the same thing. He recognized the symptoms because coincidentally his wife was suffering from the same problem so he referred me to a doctor who specialized in treating people with chemical poisoning. He diagnosed poisoning with paraquat, a weed killer used in the grounds of my workplace for the past five years coinciding with the onset of symptoms.

At last I had hope! I was treated with eight one hour sessions in a hyperbaric chamber, intravenous vitamin C and homoeopathy for the next 18 months and at the end of that time even though I was still sensitive to chemicals, medications and environmental toxins I felt well again.

As part of my recuperation, I made a number of lifestyle changes and educated myself as best I could in healthy nutrition and alternative therapies. I switched to organic food, I made my own household cleaners, got adequate rest, meditated and developed strategies for work-life balance even though it was unheard of at the time. I also saw a therapist who helped me work through the unresolved grief.

If I hadn't found the acupuncturist and the doctor who helped me I don't know how I would have survived. I was so ill I couldn't foresee another 30 or so years of my life as it had become, and there were times when I felt suicidal.

*   *   *

The recent research findings, especially those related to gene expression and brain anatomy, which demonstrate a scientific basis for 'mind over matter' effects have generated huge interest. It should be remembered, though, that investigating these topics is a complex task; that laboratory findings do not always translate into clinical practice; and that research studies which find evidence in favour of mind-body effects are much more likely to be published and quoted than others which do not. It should also be remembered that the mind-body relationship works both ways and anything wrong with the body, for example a disturbance of blood chemistry or a lesion in the brain, is likely to impact on mood and cognition. Some popular beliefs, for example that people with a positive attitude never get sick, and that being ill or failing to recover is somehow the sufferer's own fault, are over-simplistic and can cause much distress. Having a positive mindset certainly does not guarantee freedom from serious disease, nor promise recovery if disease has already developed, though it may improve the medical outlook and certainly leads to a better quality of life.

Being positive does not mean feeling obliged to fake a superficial cheerfulness which glosses over inner distress. This has been called 'the prison of positive thinking'. And it does not just mean the freedom from negativity, but is about cultivating 'high-vibration' qualities of mind such as gratitude, love, joy, hope and patience, as described later on. But before this becomes possible it is necessary to deal with the negative feelings which usually go along with being ill.

RELEASING NEGATIVE EMOTIONS

There is a vast spectrum of different feeling states, and according to some authorities these can be ranked according to their energetic frequency, with 'low-vibration' ones such as fear, guilt, sadness and despair at the bottom and 'high-vibration' ones such as love, joy, peacefulness and hopefulness at the top. Though some of the states in the middle of the range are relatively neutral, the majority can be assigned to one of two broad categories: positive ones grounded in love, and negative ones grounded in fear. Although the love-based states are more conducive to health and healing, it is often the case that the fear-based ones predominate where medical matters are concerned.

'Negative' emotions cannot, and should not, be avoided entirely. Sometimes they are appropriate to the situation, and need to be acknowledged before it becomes possible to experience genuine positive feelings. The word 'emotion' literally means 'moving outwards', and the concepts of free expression and flow are key to emotional well-being. It is the long-term persistence of negative emotional states such as grief or anger, especially when they are suppressed, which is toxic to mental and physical health.

Not only can negative emotions contribute to the development of physical disease, as discussed above, but they are a common consequence of being ill. Mental distress is an obvious and understandable response to the many depredations of physical illness: symptoms such as pain, nausea or breathlessness, restriction of activity due to weakness or immobility, concern about the future medical outcome, concern about the impact on family and finances, and direct biological effects on the structure or function of the brain.

Surveys show that a substantial minority of patients in medical settings fulfill diagnostic criteria for anxiety, depression or other mental disorder at any one time, although it is likely that many of the 'cases' identified by psychological rating scales represent appropriate responses which will only be transient, and that in the longer term these same patients will come to adjust and even experience positive psychological growth. Some however do suffer continuing distress, or develop a psychiatric illness.

It is especially important to recognise the serious condition of clinical depression, which is linked to a poor prognosis in various medical conditions, and when severe can lead to suicide. Depression can be difficult to diagnose when it coexists with physical illness, because both conditions often cause loss of appetite, weight and energy, and disturbed sleep. Mental symptoms of depression include severe and persistent sadness, lack of interest, poor concentration, feelings of guilt or worthlessness, and hopelessness about the future. Depression can often be understood as a reaction to loss, though sometimes it comes and goes for no apparent reason, and in such cases there is often a genetic element and a family history.

Anxiety, too, involves a combination of both mental and physical symptoms, illustrating the close interconnection between body and mind. When physical symptoms such as nausea, diarrhoea, breathlessness and palpitations are more prominent than mental ones, they can be confused with many different medical disorders. If a medical disorder is actually present then anxiety will make its symptoms worse, for example anxiety will exacerbate gastro-intestinal disturbances, skin conditions and almost any kind of pain. Anxiety is often worst in situations of uncertainty, such as worrying about the significance of a new symptom, awaiting diagnostic test results or preparing to undergo surgery, radiotherapy or chemotherapy. Anxiety about future health can become a long-term problem even after recovery from an episode of illness: Will I have another heart attack? Will the cancer come back? When is my next migraine attack or epileptic fit going to strike? Such fears and worries can significantly mar the enjoyment of life. Anxiety is quite understandable in these circumstances but some people, often those who have always had an anxious personality, are more vulnerable than others.

Severe depression, anxiety, and major mental disorders of other kinds require professional assessment and management, often with some combination of psychotherapy and psychotropic drugs.

Many less serious emotional problems can be successfully managed with self-help methods and CAM therapies. There are numerous different techniques to assist emotional and mental healing, for example cognitive-behavioural therapy (CBT), meditation, hypnotherapy, emotional freedom technique (EFT, tapping), homoeopathy, flower essences, energy healing, and the practice of affirmations and visualisation.

Whatever specific treatment may be used, most people who are depressed and anxious or troubled by other negative emotions will benefit a great deal from being able to talk frankly and unhurriedly about their feelings in a confidential setting, whether with a skilled professional person or with a sympathetic friend. Often, the best thing this other person can do is simply to listen attentively in a spirit of acceptance, never making judgements and seldom needing to offer advice.

Writing about painful feelings and experiences is a good alternative if there is no suitable confidant available, and those with an introverted personality may find writing easier than talking.

It is often impossible to unravel the past complexities of cause and effect as regards mind-body connections in individual people. The best approach in practice is usually to focus on the present state of mind, identifying any emotions, thought patterns, attitudes and beliefs which may be having a negative impact, with the aim of replacing these with more positive ones. No form of therapy is likely to have substantial or lasting effects unless the patient or client has enough insight and motivation to work towards change. And, to repeat, it is unrealistic to expect to feel positive all the time and 'putting on a bright face' when feeling miserable is not always a good idea. Negative feelings are part of the process of adjusting to an illness or any other adverse event, and they are better expressed than left to fester and become ingrained. It then becomes possible to move on to a genuinely positive outlook, which will improve quality of life and perhaps also improve medical outcome.

Some patients do not appear to go through a 'negative' stage at all because they are unconsciously using the mental mechanism of denial to protect themselves from fully realising the serious nature of their illness. Although complete denial can lead to problems, such as refusing a potentially helpful treatment or neglecting to organise practical affairs, partial denial can be a good way of coping and should not be challenged without good reason.

Just as darkness vanishes in the light, negative states of mind can be overcome by putting positive ones in their place. The following sections deal with some of the positive qualities which are conducive to healing.

ACCEPTANCE

People sometimes report that their illness recovered after they started accepting it as part of their lives, instead of fighting to get rid of it and striving hard to stay in control. This may seem a paradoxical effect but it could have various explanations. Resisting 'what is', because external reality does not accord with the way you want it to be, creates a great deal of stress whereas an attitude of acceptance promotes the opposite physiological state of relaxation. Acceptance also helps to make it possible to regard the illness as a friendly messenger rather than an enemy alien, and to consider that its presence may hold some meaning and purpose. These ideas will be more fully discussed later in the book.

FORGIVENESS

Inability to forgive, which includes both holding resentment towards other people and guilt towards oneself, can be highly damaging to both mental and physical health. Forgiveness is not easy, nor is it always possible or appropriate to convey it directly to the person concerned. Special techniques include expressing feelings through role play, writing them down in a letter which need not actually be sent, and 'reframing' what happened so as to bring out its more positive aspects. For example, instead of regarding themselves as a victim, the wronged person might realise that they learned something valuable from the experience or displayed great strength of character in withstanding it. Without necessarily condoning the perpetrator's behaviour, they may reach some understanding of the reasons behind it and realise that it was not necessarily intended to cause harm. One vivid personal account of the power of forgiveness comes from Greg Anderson, who had been diagnosed with terminal lung cancer but made a remarkable recovery after the expression of radical forgiveness towards a work colleague with whom he had been in conflict (www.healingcancer.info/ebook/greg-anderson).

GRATITUDE AND APPRECIATION

Turning attention towards being thankful for the good aspects of life, instead of dwelling on its problems, is a powerful way to increase happiness and well-being. Special techniques include making a mental inventory of positive things immediately after waking up in the morning, and the 'three blessings exercise' of writing down three good features of the day just gone before going to bed each night. According to the Law of Attraction, to be described later on, focusing on good things will cause them to multiply.

Appreciation is not to be confused with possessive attachment and the fear of loss.

LOVE

Love has often been described as the very essence of being, the creative energy of the universe. Love is a core value in all major religions and includes love for God, for oneself, and for everything else: other people, animals and the natural world. In New Age terminology, love is described along with peace and joy as one of the highest vibrational states. Genuine and unconditional love can dissolve the fear which underlies so much ill-health and unhappiness, and it is sometimes claimed that love and sickness cannot coexist. Many remarkable recoveries are attributed to the power of love, as described in Bernie Siegel's classic book *Love, medicine and miracles*, and in modern healing systems such as Quantum Touch (www.quantumtouch.com).

Love in its pure form is unconditional, which means it does not depend on receiving rewards and appreciation or being loved in return.

Traditionally, the part of the body most closely associated with love is the heart. Research shows that married people, especially men, live longer than those who are single, widowed or divorced (Rendall et al 2011). Loss of love, whether due to being widowed after a happy marriage or continuing to live in an unhappy marriage, is a risk factor for heart disease. Conversely, when people are 'in love' they usually enjoy enhanced well-being and relief from any health problems they may have.

Love is difficult to define and describe; it has to be felt. Thinking about a loved person or pet is one way to access the feeling. Love towards oneself is very important but, for many people, harder to experience. Louise Hay recommends frequently repeating 'I love you' in front of a mirror. Forgiveness, as described above, is a prerequisite to loving fully.

The physiological mechanisms mediating the power of love include the release of hormones such as dopamine, serotonin and oxytocin.

JOY AND LAUGHTER

Contrary to what some might expect, it is quite possible for sick people to feel joy, thereby uplifting themselves and others and promoting their bodies' self-healing powers. Happiness, contentment and pleasure are related states.

Although true joy comes from within the self rather than depending on external conditions, it is obviously easier to feel joyful if physical symptoms are well controlled, basic needs for comfort and security are met, and the surroundings are pleasant. Joy can be encouraged by loving interactions with people or animals; by helping others; by visiting a favourite place; by appreciating the beauties of nature, art or music; or by taking part in any pleasurable activity. If it is physically impossible to do such things, imagining them can help.

'Laughter therapy', 'laughter yoga' and clowning have been shown to lead to physiological benefits including lowered blood pressure, reduced stress hormone levels and improved immune function. One study found that people who smile a lot tend to live longer than their straight-faced peers. Entertainments such as watching comedy films can be a valuable distraction from the unpleasantness of illness, and may even help to improve the medical prognosis for patients with heart disease and other conditions (http://simplylaughter.com). Wholesome, innocent humour is more therapeutic than the cruel satirical kind.

Finding some humour in the illness itself can also be a good coping strategy, although this is a personal thing and some patients are easily offended by clumsy attempts to cheer them up, or by the 'black' humour which is enjoyed by many medical professionals.

HOPE

Hope is defined as 'a feeling of expectation and desire for a certain thing to happen'. According to the Law of Attraction, hope accompanied by faith can actually help the wanted outcome to manifest. The opposite of hopefulness is hopelessness, often linked to helplessness, which is established as a risk factor for morbidity and mortality from a range of conditions including cancer and heart disease. Whether 'false hope' should be challenged, for example in someone with terminal illness who appears to be denying the situation and making totally unrealistic plans for the future, is a question for debate but if mental attitude does help to shape a person's destiny it would seem important to find a balance between maintaining hope and dealing with unpleasant realities. The palliative care movement has shown that hope is both possible and therapeutic even in the most advanced cases of disease and, while 'healing is not always curing', there is always something to hope for such as better control of symptoms, rewarding relationships and activities, a peaceful death and perhaps belief in an afterlife.

PATIENCE

Being ill, or caring for someone else who is ill, demands a great deal of patience. Illness enforces slowing down, so that simple tasks of daily living take much longer to complete. A lot of time may have to be spent waiting: waiting for appointment dates, waiting in clinics, waiting for transport or caregivers to arrive at the home. Patience is also required while waiting for treatments to take effect and giving the body's own recovery processes enough time to work, for although sudden dramatic recoveries occasionally happen it is more often the case that 'healing is a process not an event' and improvement progresses slowly with setbacks along the way. Though frustrating, this can be a valuable lesson in 'living in the now', and counteracting the impatience which is endemic in modern society and is a risk factor for accidents and cardiovascular disease.

MANAGING STRESS

Stress can be defined as 'the state of physical or mental tension which results when the demands facing a person challenge their ability to cope'. This section is mainly concerned with mental stress, which affects physiology directly through secretion of 'stress hormones' such as adrenaline and cortisol. Long-term over-secretion of these hormones has been implicated in causing chronic inflammation and many physical health problems, for example high blood pressure and obesity. Stress also often leads to poor self-care, and to unhealthy behaviours such as smoking and over-indulgence in 'junk' foods, alcohol, caffeine or drugs, all of which place further stress on the body.

More than half the symptoms which people present to healthcare professionals today are believed to be primarily due to stress.

Complaints such as fatigue, poor sleep, headaches and other aches and pains, digestive and bowel disturbances often stem from this cause. Almost any medical condition is liable to be made worse by stress. However, the term 'stress' tends to be used very loosely, and it is lazy to class any illness as being 'stress-related' without specifying what is meant by stress and what other causative factors may be involved.

The stress caused by major accidents, bereavements, warfare and natural disasters is obviously severe, though it is also true that such experiences often draw out remarkable personal resources in those affected, also that the outpouring of sympathy and practical support which usually follows a shocking trauma can cushion its negative impact to some extent. Less obvious, but more common and perhaps equally harmful, is the chronic stress which many people experience in the course of their everyday lives due for example to heavy workloads, long working hours, unsatisfying work, unemployment, marital and family discord, poverty, loneliness or housing problems.

Illness itself, of course, creates stress both mentally and physically. One study (Fang et al 2012) showed that the risk of death from both suicide and cardiovascular disease increased sharply in the week following a diagnosis of cancer. It would be interesting to know whether this risk could be reduced by 'breaking bad news' in a more sensitive way and by providing more emotional support afterwards.

Though attempts have been made to rank the severity of stressful life events and difficulties in an objective fashion, it is the subjective response which really matters, and this varies tremendously between individuals due to their varying perceptions and attitudes. The same situation which causes one person to feel fear or misery may be welcomed as a challenge or relief by someone else. A great deal of stress is generated internally by high levels of anxiety or by maladaptive attitudes and beliefs.

Even when stressful circumstances cannot be altered there is always something that can be done to reduce their impact, for example learning to prioritise what is important and setting boundaries against what is not, or becoming more willing to ask for help. Revising perceptions of the situation is often possible, and this can mean accepting those things which cannot be changed rather than resisting them.

Various techniques for relieving stress are described in other parts of this book. They include mind-body practices such as relaxation and meditation; taking exercise; visiting natural surroundings; and contact with people who can offer understanding and support.

Stress cannot be avoided completely, and nor is stress altogether bad. People do need to be stretched outside their mental and physical comfort zones from time to time if they are to develop more resilience. With stress, as with so many other things in life such as alcohol and sunlight, moderation is better than too much or none at all.

RELAXATION

The word 'relaxation' as used in everyday speech can refer to anything which is perceived as leisure rather than work: for example reading, watching or playing sport, doing craftwork, making or listening to music, talking with friends, enjoying food and drink, or doing nothing at all.

The more technical use of this term refers to a physiological state called the 'relaxation response', which is the opposite of the 'stress response' described above. During the relaxation state, activity of the parasympathetic nervous system predominates over that of the sympathetic, so that the body's 'fight or flight' mode is replaced with 'growth' mode in which the cells are better able to repair themselves by absorbing nutrients and excreting the waste products of metabolism. Physically, relaxation reduces heart rate, blood pressure, rate of breathing and muscle tension. Mentally, relaxation replaces anxiety and worry with feelings of peace and calm, and improves ability to focus attention and to make decisions. Recent studies have shown that regular practice of relaxation techniques leads to beneficial changes in the expression of hundreds of the genes which are associated with health. Spending 20 or 30 minutes doing some kind of relaxation exercise each day will help to counteract the ill-effects of stress, improve sleep, and aid healing from virtually any kind of health problem, so therefore represents a good investment for anyone, sick or well.

In their book *Relaxation Revolution*, Herbert Benson and William Proctor summarise the research evidence for the benefits of relaxation, and describe how it can be used in combination with visualisation to help in the management of many specific disorders ranging from angina pectoris to premenstrual syndrome.

There are many different techniques, usually including some combination of the following:

- A 'progressive muscular relaxation' routine which involves tightening and then relaxing each group of muscles in turn,
- Deep regular breathing. Many people, especially when they are anxious, tend to take rapid shallow breaths using the upper chest alone. They therefore fail to maintain the optimum ratio between the two main gases, oxygen and carbon dioxide, involved in bodily metabolism. Breathing more slowly and deeply, using the diaphragm and abdominal muscles as well as the chest, is better,
- Mentally picturing a scene which is associated with calm and contentment.

Many different audios for guided relaxation can be downloaded from the internet, often free of charge. It is worth spending some time and effort to find the method that works best for the individual. A few people are unable to relax with any of these formal techniques, and do better by simply lying down listening to music – slow melodic music helps to regulate breathing, heart rate and blood pressure – by taking a gentle walk, or just sitting still in quiet natural surroundings and watching the clouds drift by.

Techniques for relaxation overlap with those used in meditation.

MEDITATION AND MINDFULNESS

The aim of a meditation practice is to develop calmness, compassionate detachment, and mental clarity through focus on the present moment – mindfulness.

Meditation originated as a spiritual practice in Buddhism, as the means of calming the chatter of the 'monkey mind' on the way to enlightenment. In many other religious traditions, also, meditation is used as a way of accessing the spiritual world. Most holistic healers consider a meditation practice to be an essential part of their life and work.

Meditation is also widely used, without any religious or spiritual connotations, for the purpose of stress management and in many fields of healthcare. Physiologically, meditation reduces overactivity of the sympathetic nervous system, and induces favourable neurochemical changes, characteristic EEG (electroencephalogram) patterns and, if practised regularly over time, structural changes in the brain. Thousands of studies published in recent years have shown the benefits of mindfulness in the management of many different medical conditions (Ludwig et al 2008).

There are many different schools of meditation, but the basic technique is to sit still in a quiet place, breathing gently in and out while counting the breaths, observing the thoughts and feelings and outside noises which are bound to arise but letting them drift past without getting caught up in them. This may sound simple, but most people need discipline and sustained practice to establish a routine, at least 30 minutes per day being recommended. Help is also available through modern audio technology, using music combined with subliminal sounds to induce desirable brain wave patterns.

SETTING GOALS

Defining some broad aims and specific goals can be helpful, both in relation to healing and in other domains of life. The following sections contain some direct advice about choosing goals, and using the 'manifestation techniques' of affirmation and visualisation as an aid to achieving them.

As regards the illness, you may wish to consider whether your aim is to do everything possible to achieve a cure, or whether to prioritise 'quality of life' which might mean declining certain unpleasant, risky or expensive treatments. It can also be helpful to define some measurable goals, for example increasing the number of steps you can walk each day; improving your 'numbers' on blood pressure readings or blood tests; reducing the frequency and severity of attacks of intermittent conditions such as epilepsy, migraine or asthma. Results can be recorded on written charts to monitor progress - without getting too obsessive about this, or too upset about the inevitable ups and downs.

Having other goals which are not illness-related adds meaning and enjoyment to life, and provides reason and motivation for improving health. Patients in palliative care are sometimes observed to live just long enough to reach a target date such as a family anniversary or wedding. Others might aim to complete a creative project, visit a certain place, or resolve problems in a relationship.

It is important for people to choose their own intentions and goals, rather than just going along with what others think is suitable for them. It is also important to enjoy the process, rather than being set on reaching a specific outcome within a certain time scale. Even if the intended result is achieved, which can never be guaranteed, it may feel like an anticlimax. Some authorities therefore warn against intensive pursuit of defined goals, and advise 'going with the flow' day by day, spending time on favourite activities and taking advantage of any intuitions and opportunities which may arise. With this more relaxed attitude, results may turn out even better than expected.

The achievement of goals can be aided by the techniques of affirmation and visualisation, which are based on the premise that changing your mindset can bring about changes in your physical reality, whether by means of the mind-body links discussed above or through the metaphysical workings of the Law of Attraction described later on.

AFFIRMATIONS

A positive affirmation is a statement about your desired condition. It should be phrased in the present tense as if it were already true, but not so far removed from present reality that it is impossible to believe. Saying 'My health is improving every day' would therefore be better than 'I am now in perfect health' if that is obviously not so. It is important to avoid negative statements, for example telling yourself 'I am not going to feel sick today' would not be advisable because it puts the idea of feeling sick into your mind. It is also important to be clear and unambiguous, and because it seems that words can be taken literally by 'the universe' or the subconscious mind. One woman who was under heavy pressure at work had kept repeating 'I need a break!' and then fractured a bone in her leg. Another had been saying 'I'll do anything to lose weight' for some years before she developed cancer of the stomach.

The aim is to develop a sincere belief that the affirmation is true, and feel the positive emotions which go along with that belief. Reaching this state may require the affirmations to be repeated many times each day over a period of time. Writing them down, or saying them aloud in front of a mirror, will increase their power.

Specific healing affirmations for specific medical conditions are often suggested – see for example *You can heal your life* and other books by Louise Hay – but if these do not feel right for you, feel free to write your own version. The most relevant statements are not always about the medical condition itself, but are intended to reverse the negative beliefs underlying it, for example, by encouraging love and acceptance for self and others, forgiving the past, or releasing resistance to the flow of life.

Exactly how affirmations work is not known but it has long been believed that the spoken or written word can change the structure of matter, as implied in the opening verses of St John's Gospel: 'In the beginning was the Word ... And the Word became flesh and dwelt among us'. The experiments by Masaru Emoto indicate that crystals have a more symmetrical and beautiful appearance if the water from which they were formed has been exposed to positive energies in the form of words or music. Other recent research suggests that positive affirmations can alter the expression of human DNA. Some of these studies have been criticised and are not accepted in mainstream science. There is also some evidence that positive affirmations, perhaps like most things, work better in people who already have good self-esteem.

VISUALISATION (GUIDED IMAGERY)

Visualisation techniques are based on the idea that everything exists in the emotional, mental or spiritual planes before it manifests physically. Just as a painter, architect, musician or chef conceives a mental impression of a new work before converting it into material form, the power of the mind can be used to make a template for the desired conditions. A general introduction to this topic can be found in the short book *Creative visualization* by Shakti Gawain. Visualisation can be used in medical settings to help prevent or relieve distressing symptoms, and withstand gruelling treatments, as well as to promote healing of the underlying disease. Visualisation is often combined with relaxation and affirmations, and used as part of various mind-body therapies.

One variant simply involves picturing a pleasant peaceful scene, whether based on a real memory or created in the imagination. You could distract yourself from an unpleasant situation such as lying in an MRI scanner by imagining you are in a beautiful place such as a woodland, meadow, mountain or seashore; or picture a treatment such as chemotherapy as a cleansing waterfall gently flowing through your whole being. Research carried out on patients who have practised visualisation while receiving hospital treatment for a range of conditions has shown benefits such as reduction of mental distress, easing of physical symptoms, and in some studies improved immune function and better medical outcomes. To search this topic on the internet, it is best to use the term 'guided imagery' combined with the name of the condition concerned. Some of these studies are summarised in David Hamilton's book *How your mind can heal your body*, which also includes many personal stories and practical techniques.

Specific visualisations can be used for healing purposes. For example, someone who is suffering from arthritis or recovering from an injury might picture themselves enjoying an active pursuit, such as walking or playing sport, while free from pain. Someone suffering from a skin disease might picture their skin looking smooth and perfect. Colour can be helpful here and if an inflamed body part feels like an angry red, it can be calmed by mentally infusing it with a cool blue, white or silver light.

Visualisation to strengthen the body's immune defences became a popular strategy in the cancer self-help movement some years ago after publication of the Simontons' book *Getting well again*. Some of the suggested imagery is of a militant kind, for example picturing the cells of the immune system as soldiers or sharks attacking and eliminating the unhealthy tissue. This works well for some people but others are uncomfortable with such highly aggressive images and prefer to use gentler ones, such as the sick cells quietly melting away in the presence of a pure healing light. Again, each individual will do best with an image of their own choosing. A similar approach can be used for many other medical conditions besides cancer.

Besides its application for healing purposes, visualisation can be used in relation to any other sphere of life. By creating a mental image of what you want for yourself and your surroundings, you are helping to shape your future. When you visualise, see yourself in your mind's eye enjoying a happy, active and healthy life, in as much vivid and specific detail as you can. Include sounds and scents and feelings as well as pictures. If you find it difficult to imagine something which has not happened yet, you may like to draw upon memories from the past, or look at old photographs - not in a spirit of regret, but with appreciation for the experiences you have enjoyed, so that you re-live the pleasure you felt at the time.

Though its content relates to the future and may draw upon the past, the process of visualisation is of course taking place in the present, and experiencing positive emotions while carrying it out is vital to success. As well as clearly imagining the factual details of what you desire, you need to create the good feelings you would have if it were actually happening now. This process can stimulate the release of neurotransmitters (brain chemicals) and the formation of new connections between neurons (brain cells).

KEYS TO SUCCESS WITH MANIFESTATION TECHNIQUES

There are a few more points to keep in mind, and pitfalls to avoid, when practising the 'manifestation techniques' of goal-setting, affirmation and visualisation described above.

The power of all these approaches can be increased by using a tangible format which appeals to one or more of the five senses. One method is to write a detailed description, in the present tense, of your ideal life. Assume for the purpose of this exercise that you are already in good health. Include the practicalities such as where you live and how you spend the day, your relationships, and how you want to 'be' as a person. Another method is to draw or paint a representation of what you desire; if you are not artistically inclined yourself, this can be done by combining photographs or pictures from magazines, mounted on cardboard and displayed where you will see them frequently. More sophisticated methods are available through computer technology, for example using 'mind maps' or 'mind movies'.

Whatever techniques are chosen, use them with a relaxed approach rather than striving hard to succeed. Make them fun and uplifting, so that doing them is a pleasure rather than a duty. It is not necessary to focus on them all the time, indeed this carries the danger of interfering with a process which is already underway, like digging up seeds to check on their growth. Another risk is that of giving the future too much priority over the present, so that as time slips by you will miss out on enjoying what is actually happening, and on taking advantage of other opportunities which arise. The process of living, of appreciating the good things you have already, is more important than reaching a pre-determined end point even when the present is being marred by illness. For this reason it can work well to set aside specific times periods each day to focus on the techniques, but at other times aim to 'live in the now'.

While it is good to be clear and specific about the essence of what you want, it is unhelpful to try to dictate or control all the details of when and how it will happen and exactly what the end result will be. If you remain flexible and open to the unexpected, future options which are even better than those you imagined may unfold. In any case you can never be absolutely sure of achieving the planned outcome – and even if you do, you may find it was not quite what you wanted after all. This is especially likely to happen with 'ego-based' desires which involve gaining gratification through accumulating money, possessions, or admiration from others. More real and lasting satisfaction comes from achieving those goals which fulfill your deeper values in life.

Though struggle and over-work are not recommended, you do need to play your own part in practical terms. The idea that all you have to do is affirm and imagine what you want, then simply lie back and wait for the universe to deliver it to you, is a misunderstanding. Just as there is no use dreaming about winning the lottery unless you buy a ticket, it is vital to combine these mind techniques with taking action to make positive changes in your life. If physical recovery is the aim, this means following a healthy lifestyle and taking advantage of selected treatments, as well as visualising and affirming your improved well-being.

If these techniques are so powerful, why is it that they do not always seem to work? If your condition does not improve, try not to respond with self-blame, but consider some possible reasons. First, there is usually a delay before what has been created on the vibrational plane actually manifests in material reality, and you cannot control this timing. Setting 'deadlines' for achieving your goals can create pointless stress, or force things to a premature conclusion before surrounding conditions are right. Second, material factors cannot be discounted - if an illness is very advanced and severe in biological terms it would take remarkable mental powers to reverse the process, though this is not to say that it could never be done. Third, you may be radiating mixed messages rather than pure intentions, because of internal conflicts regarding your desires and beliefs. However hard you are trying to picture yourself in radiant health, you may be holding the belief that you do not deserve to be well, or that this is not possible because you have been told your condition is incurable, or because someone else in your family had a similar illness and did not recover. Or, however sincere your desire to be healed on one level, at a deeper level you may feel afraid of being without the illness which has become such a big part of your life – for example, being well enough to return to work after a long period of sick leave can be quite a challenging prospect. Nothing in this world is all good or all bad, and even changes that are apparently positive can have anxiety-provoking aspects. So sometimes it is easier to stay with 'the devil you know', even though life with your illness is far from ideal.

As well as their self-help applications, the techniques described above form part of some professional therapies, for example hypnotherapy in which positive suggestions are presented to clients following the induction of a deeply relaxed state or 'trance'. As well as treating anxiety and other psychological problems, hypnotherapy is often effective for physical symptoms such as pain and nausea, and can help with smoking cessation. Self-hypnosis can be learned from books and audios.

MEANING AND PURPOSE IN ILLNESS

Even if an illness can be explained by a biological cause such as an infection, a toxin, an injury or a genetic mutation, it can be worth exploring deeper levels, asking what has made the person vulnerable to sickness at this particular time, and what purpose the ongoing symptoms may be serving in their life.

Illness can sometimes be understood as a 'message from the body' – or, as will be discussed in the section on spirituality, a message from the soul being conveyed through the body – that something is out of balance in the sufferer's way of 'being' or 'doing'.

This approach is meant to be a constructive one which promotes honest insight. It is not to be confused with negative beliefs about illness being a punishment for sin, or virtue being found in suffering. And it is not intended to encourage anyone to use their symptoms as an excuse to gain some kind of 'sickness benefit' in the form of financial or emotional support, or to avoid unwelcome obligations.

General interpretations which might apply to an illness of any kind include the need to rest and to be looked after following a period of stress or overwork, the need for better physical self-care, the need for more self-love and self-respect, the lack of joy and purpose in life, or just the need to be more oneself. Many people, whether or not they have consciously sought a 'message' in their illness, have found that their experience has changed some aspects of their lives for the better. One woman, after having an eye removed because of a tumour, told me 'I've lost some eyesight, but gained some insight'. She had made radical improvements to her diet, and become much more assertive in expressing her own needs rather than always complying with outside pressures: 'Learning to say no, and being strong about what was right for me in many different ways'.

More specific metaphysical meanings based on the symbolism of the symptoms, or the function of the body part involved, may be proposed. For example arthritis has been linked to a rigid and critical attitude of mind, constipation to the inability to let go of negative emotions from the past, breast cancer to a pattern of pleasing others while failing to nurture oneself, low back pain to a lack of psychological support. Correlations can be reflected in everyday speech, so that an awkward colleague might be described as 'a pain in the neck' or some unwelcome news as being 'hard to swallow'. Another theory is that one-sided ailments have a metaphysical significance, with the right side of the body being related to masculine energies and the left side to feminine ones. Interpretations based on these ideas can be over-simplistic and it is always the patient's own understanding which counts.

Looking back at the reasons for the behaviour which contributed to illness or injury can also produce insights: why did the person continue to smoke, or eat and drink too much, wear fashion shoes which damaged their feet, or get so impatient or exhausted that they had an accident?

Traditionally, orthodox medicine and psychiatry has reserved such lines of inquiry for cases in which no physical pathology could be found ('medically unexplained symptoms') or for conditions of unknown cause. The patients concerned were often dismissed as 'neurotic', 'hysterical' or even 'malingering' and sometimes referred to psychiatrists without their knowledge or consent. Conversely, for cases in which a respectable 'organic disease' had been diagnosed, important psychological aspects were ignored. Peptic ulcer, for example, used to be classed as a 'psychosomatic' condition requiring psychotherapy but after *Helicobacter pylori* was identified as a causative agent, purely physical treatment became the norm and the stress-related aspect received little further attention even though it was often significant (Levenstein 1998). Hopefully this kind of dichotomous thinking is becoming replaced by a more neutral and compassionate approach which acknowledges that mind and body are closely interconnected and that all illness is in some sense 'psychosomatic'.

PART 4

The Spiritual Level

The term 'spiritual' is often defined by exclusion as referring to that which is not material or physical. 'Spirit', often spelled with a capital 'S', can be understood as the intangible vital force or energy which creates and sustains life in all its forms. If the spiritual realm governs the physical one, everything exists as a spiritual blueprint before it materialises in physical form. The spiritual aspect of an individual person can be described as their 'soul', 'Higher Self' or 'spirit' with a small 's'.

Serious illness often prompts exploration of spiritual and existential questions, for example whether there is meaning in suffering, whether there is a God and whether there is life after death.

According to a number of research studies, spiritual awareness and belief in some kind of higher power tend to be good for health, although concepts like these can only be partly captured by means of questionnaires and statistical analyses. Spiritual awareness does not necessarily include affiliation to a formal religion, although it has been shown that membership of a church or other religious organisation is beneficial to health in its own right. This is probably because, as well as having direct spiritual benefits, it promotes a regular lifestyle and provides a network of social support. This section of the book is not concerned with formal religion but mainly with the so-called New Age spirituality which is embraced by a majority of holistic healers. The spiritual and the psychological aspects of being cannot always be separated and so some of the material here overlaps with that in Part 3 above.

The concept of spirit is often rejected by atheists and rationalists, including many conventional scientists. However, there is evidence from modern quantum physics that what appears to be empty space between atomic particles is actually a field of energy and information, pervading everything in the universe, and transcending time and space. Though described in very different terminology, this field could well be equivalent to the concept of God or Divine Intelligence which is recognised in all the world's religions, and is in keeping with the concept of 'subtle energies' described below.

THE SUBTLE ENERGY MODEL

Holistic healers consider the balance and flow of energy as being crucial to health and disease. Descriptions of the human organism as an energy system date back to the ancient mystical traditions of the East. This type of energy has been called 'subtle' because it is not detectable with conventional measuring instruments. Though many Western clinicians would consider this paradigm alien and bizarre, it is being increasingly validated by discoveries in modern science (Kelly 2011), and it has been suggested that 'energy medicine' is the way of the future and will replace the older mechanical and chemical approaches (Dossey 1999). A brief summary of the main concepts now follows.

All that exists in the physical universe is created from a vast field of energy and information which permeates and interconnects both animate and inanimate things, human beings included. The manifestations of this field are influenced by human consciousness and it is 'non-local', not being limited by time or space. This would explain such phenomena as telepathy, distant healing and the influence of prayer.

Living beings are animated by a 'vital force' also called chi, qi or prana.

The human organism is composed of concentric layers of energy which vibrate at different frequencies. The physical body, the densest layer, is surrounded by a 'biofield' in the form of an aura, which can be seen by clairvoyants and felt by sensitive people, recorded by Kirlian photography and viewed by a number of more modern instruments. Though the existence of this complex electromagnetic field is often denied in orthodox circles, it was formally acknowledged by the U.S. National Institutes of Health in 1994. The aura is said to contain seven main layers, with the innermost or etheric layer being like a template which shapes and informs the physical body. The outer layers, each with progressively higher vibrations, are concerned with the psychological and spiritual aspects of being. All the layers are interconnected with each other and with the wider universe. Therefore the spirit, or soul, of each human being is connected with those of other beings and with the wider Spirit, or Source.

The energy centres called chakras are like spinning wheels placed parallel to the spine along its length. Each of the seven main chakras is related to one or more colours of the rainbow, aspects of psychology, endocrine glands and local organs. For the fourth chakra, for example, these are green and rose pink; love and compassion; thymus, heart, lungs and breasts. This chakra is also known as the heart chakra and merits special significance if, as recent research suggests, it is the heart rather than the brain which is the seat of emotion and intuition and the main portal of communication with the universal energy field (www.HeartMath.org). Another example is the fifth, or throat, chakra which is associated with the colour blue and is concerned with communication and self-expression.

In Chinese medicine, energies are divided into 'yin' and 'yang', the passive feminine and the active masculine principles, which ideally need to be fairly equally balanced with one another in persons of either sex.

According to the holistic model, a balanced and coherent flow of energies in the biofield is a prerequisite for good health. In contrast, if there is a blockage or depletion of subtle energies at the psycho-spiritual levels, well-being is reduced and the body is rendered more vulnerable to disease-causing agents. This would be consistent with the observations from many modern research studies that negative psychological states, such as depression and loneliness or experience of traumatic events, are significant precursors of morbidity and mortality, even if the postulated mechanisms are quite different. Besides individual personal factors, disruptions in the subtle energies could arise from changes in earth energies or planetary cycles, or trends in mass consciousness. Whether through the perceptions of a sensitive person or clairvoyant, or by reading images from a biofield viewing machine, it may be possible to pick up disruptions in the human energy field which could lead to disease later on.

'Vibrational medicines' such as acupuncture, homoeopathy, flower essences, colour therapy and the many forms of energy healing are designed to correct imbalances in the energy field (Gerber 2000).

SPIRITUAL AND ENERGY HEALING

The word 'healing' has been used throughout this book in its general sense to mean restoring health, wholeness and balance. 'Healing' is also a short-hand term for the group of therapies called spiritual healing or energy healing. Spiritual healers work by focusing their intention on the highest good of their clients and entering into an altered state of consciousness in which their own intellect and emotions are put aside and they become channels through which the universal higher energies can flow. Studies show that the electromagnetic radiation emitted from their bodies increases during this process.

To quote from the website of the College of Healing (www.collegeofhealing.org, accessed 2013):

'Healing is the offering of universal energy with the specific aim of restoring a state of balance to the healee on all levels, physical, emotional, mental and spiritual.

'The key is that healing should always be given as an offering of unconditional love, with an approach of "thy will be done". It is not for the healer to determine what the client's spirit needs or desires, however they may use their skills to help the client to achieve their own state of balance within any given circumstance.

'Healing can be of great value in a variety of different situations, as it allows the client to regain their own sense of balance and harmony. It is by assisting the client with the removal of blockages to their energetic system and bringing their system back into balance that the healer is able to help the client to achieve the changes they desire. These changes can happen on every level of the client's system - physical, emotional, mental and spiritual.'

Broadly speaking there are two types of spiritual healing: contact healing and distant healing. With contact healing, practitioners use their hands to assess, balance and strengthen their clients' energy fields. They usually work several inches away from the body without actually touching it. People who receive healing often enter a deeply relaxed state. They may feel warmth, cold or tingling, see colours or images, hear music or smell scents.

With distant healing the clients are not physically present, and the process appears to work just as well as contact healing, even from the other side of the world. There are reports of distant healing having an effect when it is carried out without the sick person's knowledge, and laboratory studies have demonstrated changes in EEG and fMRI when people are receiving distant healing but do not know it is taking place .

Just as a radio or TV can only receive certain frequencies if it is tuned appropriately, healing can only work for those who are open to accepting it, though this does not necessarily need to be at conscious level.

The specific outcome of any healing interaction is unpredictable, because the process involves surrendering to the grace of a higher power rather than the exercise of personal control by either healer or client. Occasionally there will be a rapid and complete recovery from disease. More often there is a gradual improvement, which does not necessarily result in a cure but includes lessening of symptoms and greater peace of mind. Almost all clients experience something positive from healing sessions and the majority of clinical research studies have reported a favourable effect (Benor 2007). Again quoting from the College of Healing website:

'The aim of healing is to create a space of balance for the individual; this is not necessarily the same as cure. The side effects of this space of balance and healing may be cure from the illness or disease; alternatively there may be a new attitude within the individual on how to deal with their circumstance. The healer's task is to use their skills to create the space for the individual to enable their own healing, rather as a physician would create the space for mending a broken leg by applying a plaster cast, but it is the individual's own leg that heals itself. It may, for example, be the individual's spiritual wish to experience the disease in full, and not to be cured in the conventional sense, nevertheless, by giving healing, the healer may be able to affect a change in the mental, or emotional state of the client which allows them to deal better with their disease process. Healers should never impose their own will, be this for cure or any other area, onto the client.'

Healing is also beneficial for healers themselves. Rather than draining their own personal resources, it involves them in a positive exchange and renewal of energy. However, just like anyone else working in a caring profession, they need to look after themselves well and maintain their own sources of support.

All healers believe in the spiritual realm, and some are affiliated with particular religions. The Christian healing ministry is based on the miracles performed by Jesus, who cured many people from a wide variety of mental and physical ailments. Other healers work with different religious traditions, or with the New Age spirituality which has no fixed dogma but draws upon various faiths and philosophies. Essentially, it includes trust in a higher energy of goodness and love, which unites all forms of life – humans, other animals, plants and the Earth itself. Healers may invoke spirit guides or angels, and combine their work with other modalities such as counselling, visualisation, colour therapy or crystal therapy. The many specialised forms of healing including Reiki, Reconnective Healing, Quantum Healing and Therapeutic Touch. While just a few people possess a natural healing gift, anyone who is sincerely motivated can learn to practise these methods.

PRAYER (Dossey 1993)

Prayer has been defined as 'a reverent petition to God or an object of worship'. Remarkable recoveries are occasionally observed following prayers for healing, whether carried out by sick people themselves, or through the intercession of others praying on their behalf with or without their knowledge. However, there are limits to what can be achieved, for example I do not believe there are any recorded cases of missing limbs growing back again. Also, the effect of prayer upon prognosis is unpredictable. Not all illnesses will recover and, after all, everyone has to die one day. For this reason, though some authorities advise praying for a specific outcome, others say it may be best just to ask for the patient's 'highest good'.

The formal evidence about the effects of prayer on recovery from illness is conflicting. Early studies suggested a benefit, but this was not confirmed by a large randomised trial in which patients having coronary artery bypass graft surgery who knew that they were being prayed for actually suffered a higher rate of complications than those who were either not receiving prayers, or did not know whether they were or not (Benson, Dusek, Sherwood et al 2006). Inevitably, studies on this topic involve a contrived situation very different from the real-life one in which sick individuals may receive prayers from their own family and friends. It could also be questioned whether it is ethical to pray for some patients but not for others on the basis of randomisation.

THE LAW OF ATTRACTION

Practices such as visualisation, affirmation and goal-setting, already discussed in Part 3, involve not only mental techniques but also the metaphysical concept known as the 'Law of Attraction' (LOA). According to this, 'like attracts like' because everything in the universe is made up of energy, and energies of similar vibrational frequency are drawn together. The energetic vibrations generated by people's thoughts, attitudes, beliefs, emotions, intentions and focus of attention resonate with corresponding frequencies in the surrounding universe and magnetise them into their life experience.

The LOA has been known for centuries, though not necessarily under that name, and its principles can be recognised in many ancient religions and philosophies as well as in modern self-help writings. Comprehensive information can be found through the Abraham-Hicks website (www.abraham-hicks.com), CDs and books. The 2006 movie called *The Secret* provided a more simplistic, and some would say too materialistic, exposition which became widely known.

In general terms, a negative mindset would attract unwanted experiences such as that of illness whereas a positive one would attract desirable ones including good health. More specifically, sustained mental concentration on a certain topic would eventually cause it to materialise. I am not aware of any formal evidence for this effect in terms of disease states, but have known several cardiologists who had heart attacks, oncologists who developed cancer, and psychiatrists who committed suicide. Obviously nobody would deliberately want to attract ill-health in this manner, but they might do so unwittingly by thinking about it too much, whether in the context of their professional work or through sustained worry about their personal risk.

The deliberate, conscious application of the LOA can be summed up in the three steps 'Ask, Believe, Receive'.

'Ask': this requires being clear about what it is you want and it needs to be phrased in positive terms, as already discussed in the section on Affirmations in Part 3. Many people fail to get the results they desire because they are focusing on what they do not want rather than what they do want. Asking 'not to have arthritis in my knees' puts the mental focus on what is unwanted and could have the opposite effect. A positive alternative would be 'To be able to walk freely'.

'Believe': this is about having faith, and generating the positive emotion that you would be feeling if your wish had already been fulfilled. If this seems too much like self-delusion, think of your vividly-imagined desire already existing at the energetic level, in what Abraham-Hicks calls your 'vibrational escrow', just waiting to manifest in the physical realm. The practice of visualisation, already described in Part 3, is relevant here.

'Receive': it is claimed that if you 'ask' and 'believe' in the right way your desires will inevitably be granted, though maybe not for some time, nor in quite the way you envisaged. Sometimes, what we think we want is not actually what would be best for us in the long term. In any case, there is usually a delay in manifestation. This allows leeway to reconsider any sudden impulses which were misguided, or for the surrounding circumstances to line up so that everything happens at the best time.

If you have been told that you have a progressive incurable disease, and are continually experiencing symptoms which remind you of this, it is far from easy to create a convincing alternative reality through your imagination. But many people have done it, and reported recovery from serious conditions through use of this technique.

The 'ask, believe, receive' formula needs to be combined with practical action for best results.

EXPLORING SPIRITUAL ORIGINS OF ILLNESS

The idea that illness can carry a psychological message regarding imbalance in a person's outlook or way of life was discussed in Part 3. This concept can be taken further if the spiritual dimension is added.

The human soul is believed to be immortal, existing before birth and surviving after death, and according to many belief systems ranging from Ancient Greek philosophy to the New Age movement of today each person's spirit carries an intention for their incarnation on planet Earth. The circumstances of their life will be chosen by their spirit guides to assist them in fulfilling a certain purpose, or learning certain lessons which will advance their spiritual growth. They may veer off their intended path if there is a misalignment between their earthly personality (ego) and their Higher Self (soul). Practical examples of this may be seen in those doctors, lawyers and other professionals whose soul's calling to serve their patients or clients has become over-ridden by their ego's craving to make as much money as possible in private practice. An illness can sometimes be the stimulus for getting back on track. These ideas are clearly explained in the classic short book Heal thyself by Edward Bach, the doctor who discovered the Bach flower remedies.

Other, more controversial theories about the spiritual origins of illness involve beliefs about reincarnation, spirit possession, and the collective consciousness. These are somewhat beyond the scope of this book but will be briefly considered here.

Many traditions teach that the soul goes through repeated incarnations on its journey towards enlightenment. There are reported cases in which the present symptoms appear to correspond with a trauma from a previous lifetime, as recalled either spontaneously or through hypnotic regression. An example would be a skin lesion at the site of a previously fatal injury. Bizarre as this phenomenon may seem to the Western scientific mind, it gains some credence from systematic studies such as those by the psychiatrists Ian Stevenson and Jim Tucker, based on thousands of interviews with young children who claimed to remember past lives. Discussions about reincarnation often include the concept of karma, a universal law which is concerned with the balancing of energy, as summed up in the phrase 'what goes around comes around'. So, a person who inflicted pain on others in a former life might suffer pain themselves in a later incarnation.

The idea behind spirit possession is that the spirit of somebody who was troubled at the time of death has been unable to make the usual transition to the other side, but remains 'earthbound' and attaches itself to a vulnerable person, causing mental or physical illness, substance addiction or various other problems in life. Suspected cases have sometimes been successfully treated by 'spirit release therapy' or religious exorcism.

As regards the collective consciousness, the theory is that the prevalent beliefs and attitudes of groups of people – whether within families, or particular cultures, or the human race as a whole – act to magnify the energies which can affect health. Fear and hate in general would tend to generate illness, and there could be more specific correlations with particular symptoms or diseases. In contrast, love and compassion would support health. It is the more sensitive and empathic individuals within the group who are most vulnerable to these effects, so becoming the 'carriers' of other people's problems, acting as vehicles for manifesting negativity which originated outside themselves. Examples of this can be seen when healers 'take on' the same symptoms as their clients, especially when they have not paid enough attention to looking after themselves well and maintaining their own personal boundaries.

The theories outlined above are most likely to be invoked for cases of illness which cannot be explained in any other way and have failed to respond to the usual treatments. It may be impossible to research them through the methods of conventional science, however this does not necessarily mean that they are invalid. Some people find them helpful, while others do better to accept that the cause of their illness is simply not known. I believe it is best to keep an open mind about spiritual theories without getting so carried away as to ignore physical causes and treatments.

AUTHENTICITY

Authenticity, accepting and being true to one's own nature, is an important aspect of maintaining or recovering good health. It includes expressing emotions more openly, focusing on interests and goals more clearly, not relying too much on outside opinions, and living in closer accordance with personal values. Personal values are qualities and concepts, mostly of an abstract nature: examples include freedom, concern for justice, contribution to others, appreciation of beauty, creativity, adventure, connections with family and friends, and the pursuit of knowledge.

One of the chief regrets expressed by people with a terminal illness is 'I wish I'd had the courage to live a life true to myself, not the life others expected of me' (Ware 2012).

Authentic people follow their own path in life without too much regard for external rewards such as money, praise or fame. In contrast, those who habitually suppress their own needs and desires, due to an exaggerated sense of duty or a craving for approval, frequently end up feeling resentful and may become physically unwell.

In her book *Practical miracles*, Arielle Essex proposes that unless you are clear about who you are and where you want to go in life, it will be difficult for the trillions of cells in your body to work together in harmony or for your immune system to distinguish 'self' from 'non-self'. There are certainly many stories of improvements in health following a change to a more authentic way of being. In his book *Cancer as a turning point*, Laurence LeShan stresses the importance of 'singing your own song' in life and includes many case histories to show how this can lead to healing. Healing does not always mean curing, as illustrated by the following case history which relates to a woman in her 60s who was a personal friend of mine. It was her wish to contribute to this book and with her permission I have included aspects of her story both below and in Part 6, quoting extracts from the various emails which she sent me during her illness.

This woman had been feeling extremely tired for several weeks before noticing a swelling in her neck. A biopsy showed this to be a lymph node containing secondary tumour deposits from a cancer of the mouth. She had always followed a healthy lifestyle and did not have any of the known physical risk factors for this disease, but felt that it could be linked to having 'kept her mouth shut' for many years while living in an unsatisfactory marriage, and more recently having felt unable to tell her husband about her relationship with another man. This relates to the idea that blockage of communication and self-expression is related to disease of the organs governed by the fifth chakra. Not everyone would accept this explanation as valid, but it proved liberating to her, and following the cancer diagnosis she found the courage to tell her husband the true situation, and soon afterwards moved in to live with her new partner. She wrote 'It feels so freeing and right to be following one's own path and living true to self. … the rough bits have been ROUGH and I know we have more difficult decisions ahead … but we are VERY SURE we want each other and so we are just getting through it.' Sadly she did not recover from the cancer, but she found great happiness in her new relationship during the final months of her life.

An illness can be like a signpost which points to a new way forward and though the old way may have been blocked, or no longer feels right, something different and better is revealed.

EXPLORING LIFE PURPOSE

However long or short a life may be, having a sense of purpose can make it seem more worthwhile.

Questions about life purpose, whether for the human race in general or for the individual seeking personal fulfillment, have been discussed in philosophical and religious circles since ancient times and are also a focus of many personal development systems today. Although there may be no definitive answers to such questions, there are many suggestions about how to approach them. One simple formula which can be helpful is:

Passion + Mission = Purpose.

'Passion' is what you love to do, and 'Mission' is how you can use it for the benefit of others, so 'being the best you can be'.

Most people do not have a clear idea about their main passion or mission, and it may be that individual life purpose is best viewed as a multi-faceted and flexible concept which unfolds as time goes on but may always remain something of a mystery.

Even if the 'big picture' is unseen, it is helpful to have some general intentions and specific goals. Expressing interests and talents, following intuitions, being aware of synchronicities such as apparent coincidences and chance happenings, and seeking the 'message' in adverse events such as illness, can provide clues to direction and perhaps eventually fit together like pieces of a jigsaw as discussed in my own ebook *Life's labyrinth*.

SPIRITUALITY IN NATURE

Besides providing physical benefits such as breathing fresh air, taking exercise, being exposed to sunlight and connecting with the earth, time spent out of doors in natural surroundings is spiritually uplifting. Observing the beauty of a flower or sunrise, the rhythm of the tides, the peace of a forest or the majesty of a mountain can inspire a sense of wonder and of oneness with all creation.

Even those who are not well enough to go outside can benefit from having plants in their rooms, or from viewing natural scenery. One study showed that surgical patients who could see trees from their hospital windows recovered more quickly than those who looked out on bare walls (Ulrich 1984). Sadly, many hospital environments are divorced from nature, and when anxious patients and hard-pressed staff are crowded together in stark surroundings with high levels of noise, bright lights and radiation, the atmosphere is likely to be stressful rather than healing. This situation can be improved to some extent if wards are decorated with calming colours such as green and blue.

CREATIVITY

Creativity can be defined as the expression of imagination and originality, and is by no means limited to the traditional creative arts of writing, music, painting and craftwork. Raising a family, starting a business or developing a home and garden are examples of creativity in its broadest sense. Life itself can be considered a creative journey, and anyone can live creatively by putting their individual stamp on their chosen activities, and making the most of their unique combination of interests, talents and values. Blockage of creative expression has often been proposed as a contributing factor in illness, as in the famous line by the poet WH Auden implying that cancer could be a consequence of 'foiled creative fire'.

Illness can act as a stimulus to creativity in a number of ways. Some people are able to develop their creative side after being ill simply because they have more time available. Physical limitations permitting, being off work and confined to the home might be an opportunity to take up writing, drawing, cooking, knitting, gardening, or playing a musical instrument.

The illness itself can be a source of material for creative work, and many professionals have gained inspiration in this way. The Mexican artist Frida Kahlo used vivid images and colours to portray her suffering after spinal injury in paintings such as *The broken column*. The Russian writer Alexander Solzhenitsyn drew upon his own experience as a patient for his novel *Cancer ward*. The visual aura which precedes attacks of classical migraine has inspired many pieces of art. In addition to having technical merit, and hopefully being therapeutic for the artists themselves, works like this can help to educate and inform the public about the realities of illness.

The healing benefits of the creative arts can be absorbed in a passive way by appreciating other people's work. Actively creating something original has a still more powerful effect. This is nothing to do with making something 'good' for public display. Its essential value lies in private self-expression, which can help with adjustment and coping and aid the recovery process. Healing through the creative arts is available to anyone, whether or not they have any special talents and skills in these fields, and whether or not they wish to share the results with others. Two well-researched modalities, which can be explored either alone or with the guidance of a therapist, are music and art.

Research studies have shown that simply listening to music has many positive effects on health - benefits include the relief of pain from many causes, improved sleep, reduced anxiety, enhanced mental development in children, and more rapid recovery of memory following a stroke. Actively singing or playing an instrument, as opposed to passive listening, brings in many other positive factors and professional music therapy, which involves sophisticated techniques adapted for each client, can have still more powerful effects.

Music works to promote healing in many different ways. At the physical level, appropriately chosen music can help to regulate various aspects of physiology, and encourage formation of new neural connections in the brain. Different sound frequencies have specific effects. The vibration of a cat's purr, for example, is conducive to bone and tissue repair. Some biofeedback devices work through sound frequencies individually selected to modify the client's symptoms. The 528 Hz frequency, found in the 6-note Solfeggio scale, has been called the 'frequency of love' and some claim it has special healing power, enabling DNA to absorb ultraviolet light and attune the body's rhythm to that of the cosmos. It is found in many of the old Gregorian chants, and is featured in various modern videos which can be found on YouTube.

At the emotional level, music is a channel for the expression of feelings which are beyond words, and can enable deep sadness or anger to be released. Many of us have poignant memories associated with particular pieces and therefore the choice of music, and the meaning attached to it, is always specific to the individual concerned. Music has a spiritual element too, and plays an important part in the services and rituals of most religious traditions. Other benefits of music, which I have personally experienced since I joined a choir some years ago, include the social aspects of singing or playing instruments in a group, and the mental exercise of studying music theory. Music, therefore, carries a wide range of potential rewards and must be rated as among the most valuable of all aids to the healthy integration of body, emotions, mind and spirit.

Art employs a different channel of creativity. In art therapy, the spontaneous choice of images and colour can enable feelings to be made conscious, expressed and transformed. A picture of a wild animal or bird of prey, or of a tree being buffeted and broken in a storm, might represent a sick person's feelings of being under attack by their illness. On a more positive note, a sunrise over the sea or a flower in a desert might symbolise new beginnings or the dawning of hope. Talking with an art therapist can help to clarify the meaning of what has emerged, and painting a series of pictures over time can facilitate an emotional journey. Some beautiful and striking works have been produced in the art therapy setting, and these may convey a graphic sense of the illness experience if made available for public view. Again, however, many clients would prefer to keep their artwork private, and they must be assured that the aim is to improve their own well-being rather than to develop technical expertise or put on a show.

TRANSFORMATIONAL RESPONSES

The idea that health problems can carry a message has been a recurring theme in this book. Sometimes the message is a simple practical one, such as needing to take more rest or drink more water. Sometimes the body part involved, or the specific nature of the symptoms, holds a symbolic significance. Sometimes the experience of being sick has a deeper spiritual impact, and ultimately proves life-enhancing. I do not want to over-state these positive aspects, because all illnesses involve suffering, and it does not always ring true to hear them described as 'a gift' or 'a wake-up call' - especially by people who have never been seriously ill themselves. But there is often some truth in these clichés – and in the old proverb 'every cloud has a silver lining'.

Many survivors of serious illness report greater appreciation of life, closer relationships, and a clearer sense of what is important to them, with less concern about material possessions: 'I feel strangely free of "things" and able to live without my books, china etc'. And a minority undergo a truly 'transformational response' in which major changes in their ways of 'being' and 'doing' lead to a more purposeful rewarding and authentic life. Some would express this as the earthly personality becoming better aligned with the soul, or Higher Self. This process is sometimes, but by no means always, accompanied by physical healing.

One truly inspiring description of transformation can be found in Anita Moorjani's book *Dying to be me*. Following a near-death experience (NDE), she not only recovered from apparently terminal lymphoma, but underwent profound changes in her outlook on life. In her book she is careful to avoid dogma, emphasising that every path to healing is different, however the principles which she describes – which include living from love rather than fear, recognising the divine perfection and magnificence of all beings, being true to yourself and loving yourself, being present in the now, and having fun - are surely of universal value. Many others have reported similar experiences following an NDE, and thousands of personal accounts can be found on the website www.nderf.org.

It is of course possible to undergo a personal transformation without having such a momentous experience as an NDE, though the effect is seldom so radical or sudden. And it is not always necessary or desirable to undergo drastic change in order for lasting healing to occur. On the other hand, wanting life to go back to exactly the way it used to be may not be such a good idea, because this means replicating the conditions under which the illness developed in the first place.

The following account describes a gradual awakening of spirituality and creativity, and a positive change of life path, after finding the 'message' in an accident. It was contributed by Liz Gunning, who lives and works in her family's fine arts centre in Shropshire, England (www.ironbridgeframing.co.uk) and who, like me, is a graduate of the College of Healing (www.collegeofhealing.org).

LIZ'S STORY

It was a bright sunny day; the men were working well repairing the roof of our Victorian house. So Dave and I decided to take the puppies for an early morning stroll across the meadow. I felt a light spring to my step, as I had completed all my schemes of work for the next term's lessons.

Walking along the road I suddenly heard a cracking of branches – but the only thing was - the sound came from within my right leg. I calmly said 'I think I've broken my leg, Dave' and with that I seemed to glide to the ground, suddenly feeling the surge of pain hitting me as my foot dislocated behind me as I impacted with the harsh road surface.

From that moment on, my life flashed in front of me. I seemed to see windscreen wipers swishing one way and another. As they moved so did the gush of pain pulse through my body, and voices were whispering telling me to 'Let go' in a repeated motion in time with the windscreen wipers.

I knew in an instant my teaching career was over and also that this was fate! I had been so unhappy at school, almost to burnout situation. Our two mums had both died some four months back and we were still recovering from the awful shock of those sad weeks.

Whilst lying on the hard tarmac I could hear the whispers of the Angels in my ears telling me to let go, and I couldn't do anything other – I couldn't move – I was completely at the mercy of the elements.

On arrival at the hospital, I was waiting to have my ankle pulled back into position (it was completely dislocated, and I had broken both my tibia and fibula) when in came three men who approached me with determined looks on their faces. They began pulling at my leg and foot and telling me to hold still. The pain was so great, until I was suddenly transported into the most wonderful flight over the Ironbridge Gorge. I really was flying, I wasn't in pain and I was soaring with the doves over the River Severn. It was beautiful. But then I felt sucked back into my body like a whirlwind as I felt the surging pain yet again thumping through my body like a tidal wave. I knew I was in for the long haul! I came to as a big wet bandage was being wrapped around my poor leg. My husband looked as white as a sheet!

There was one more trip to A & E where my foot completely gave way; and the Doctor I saw grabbed it with such vigour that I hit out with the pain. 'Ah, ah,' he exclaimed, 'You have CRPS (Chronic Regional Pain Syndrome). You really are in pain, aren't you?'

I attended a 'Pain Management Course' and it was on this that I was first introduced to emotional issues to do with my foot! It wasn't until then that I began to realise just how my emotions were impacting on the other elements of my body. For me, the key to repairing my foot was repairing my life, which meant delving into the past to sort out my emotions about my family, my job and my physical well being.

I had been an art teacher for many years and enjoyed the challenge of passing on my knowledge to young children in a practical and caring manner. I was given great recognition for this and gained many accolades for the schools I worked for. I had however become 'burnt out' by giving too much, and did not listen to my inner voice saying 'It's time to change your life, Liz, this job is preventing you from moving forwards! Let go!' The consequence was that my exhaustion impacted on me physically and down I came, to a complete halt. I had to let go whether I liked it or not.

One year later I eventually had the pins and plates removed from my leg (the nuts were lose and I could see them wobbling!) and I still couldn't weight-bear. No one except my husband believed that I was still in excruciating pain. Healing helped and during my visits to my psychotherapist, Annie, I began to find I was able at times to put the pain to one side.

Intuitively I began occupying my time with my ceramics, and fleetingly said to Annie on one of my visits that I was away with the fairies when centring clay on the potter's wheel.

She asked, 'Does that mean you are in no pain when sitting on the potter's wheel?'

'Yes, Annie, it's wonderful. I feel so free, no pain, no stabbing feelings from the base of my foot. It's wonderful.'

With that information I really began the journey of learning how to use the energies of my body to help heal my wounds. I became a student again at the tender age of 53, and passed the Basic Healing Course with the College of Healing. This taught me how to centre myself (just the same as on the potter's wheel) and how to meditate to allow peace to be felt from within. Sometimes when I meditated I was joined by a whopping big beautiful wild hare. Consequently, I sculpted a four-foot hare out of local sandstone and he now proudly sits in our front garden overlooking the Ironbridge Gorge. I was able to side-step the pain when sculpting this hare, he is quite a beauty I must admit! Again all part and parcel of my healing process.

I learned, over time, how to resume family life without referring to 'the foot' and realized just how much influence the Angels had in helping me re-shape my life.

I met Claudia, a clairvoyant, who instantly exclaimed that I had an Angel standing right by my side. She told me the Angel was there for me as my guide and my helper through my trials with learning how to walk again.

I began, with Annie's superb help, healing the traumas of my life and realised just how much my family had held me back during my childhood years. I learnt to recognise the impact on my body and how to centre and ground myself on a daily basis.

It wasn't easy, after all I was still human, and at times anger took over with me lashing out 'Why me!'

My teaching career was by now well and truly over. This I didn't mind as I intuitively knew I was on another pathway. The Angels kept the whispering going 'Let go, Liz, and allow yourself just to be!'

Again easier said than done as the pain would surge as the bed clothes gently contacted with my scars, and as for going swimming, well no chance, the water swishing and making contact with my foot was just purgatory. The daggers still penetrated up through my foot as I walked but somehow I began to accept rather than thrash. I was learning to 'Let Go'.

I still continued healing the childhood wounds and began to understand the real me! I was a good person, dedicated to my job and of value to society. The knots in my stomach began to disentangle as I began learning the finer art of the chakras and the aura that surrounded me.

Colour plays an important part in my life as a potter and as a family rooted in the arts, and I began to see my chakras as pure colour wheels spinning brightly from within, and as the months rolled into years so I began to improve in my walking ability and so my life became so much brighter.

I began the Diploma Course with the College of Healing and this pushed me further into my intuitive healing skills. Every essay I wrote I enjoyed, I was switching on my brain to new and amazing things like earth energies, meditation, and doorkeepers and guides. All new and exciting phenomena that resonated so well with my heart. The emotions I have felt and the experiences I have encountered have led me into new and wondrous pathways.

I have stumbled, if you like, and been given a new pathway to follow. One whereby others have helped me to heal and in doing so I too am becoming a healer – a Wounded Healer. Healing energy flows when hearts connect, and the Wounded Healer understands what the patient feels because he or she has gone through the same pain.

It has taken nearly seven years to repair and still I'm in pain, however the pain has changed, I'm proud of it when it sparks as it's a reminder of the journey I have travelled with the Angels. I am able to swim with my grandchild on a regular basis; I can dig the garden, stride out over the meadows and landscapes of Shropshire where I live knowing my inner self is happy and content.

I must thank my dear Husband, Dave for being with me every step of the way (excuse the pun), my two loving daughters Sarah and Jenny, my son-in-law Nathan and of course my Psychotherapist, Annie. What a woman! What a journey!

PART 5

Healing Relationships

SUPPORT FROM FAMILY AND FRIENDS

The quality of relationships with partners and families, friends and workmates, healthcare professionals and fellow patients can have a direct effect on health, besides being important as regards coping with illness. Therefore it is highly desirable to replace 'toxic' relationships with supportive ones wherever possible.

Supportive personal relationships provide both emotional and practical benefits. People with strong 'social networks' tend to have lower morbidity and mortality than those who live in isolation. Married people, especially men, tend to have better health and live longer than the single, widowed or divorced (Rendall et al 2011). These associations have been especially well researched for heart disease (Bunker et al 2003), and can be partly explained by physiological mechanisms (Uchino 2006).

Having a partner, family and friends who are loving and sympathetic, and able to provide daily assistance and care, is obviously of great benefit to a sick person. Conversely, difficult relationships may impede coping and recovery. If a relationship has been problematic all along, the stress of illness often makes things worse. Some partners and family members are unable to face the situation and opt out, either emotionally or in practical ways. Others, while appearing to help and often genuinely believing that they are helping, take over total control and so deprive patients of the last vestiges of choice and independence. It is easy to blame the healthy partners in such situations, but carers have an exhausting and demanding part to play and they may be suffering just as much as the patients themselves, though in different ways.

Conflicted relationships can be worse than none at all and for someone who feels trapped in a stifling or abusive partnership, healing may be impossible unless and until they can muster the courage and practical resources to leave. However, such a radical solution is only necessary in a few cases. More often, relationships are a mixture of good and bad, and rather than ending them completely it is a question of making changes to improve them. Carers may need more support for themselves. Patients may need to be assertive enough to set firmer boundaries and to express their needs more openly. This could mean explaining to other people what they can do or say to help, and pointing out things which are not helpful, such as making gloomy predictions about prognosis or taking over their roles without being asked. All those involved can benefit from learning to say 'no' to unwelcome requests, and from arranging to spend some protected time alone for self-care, self-development and relaxation.

Difficult relationships can always be a 'learning experience'. Some would say that they represent the working out of karma from previous lifetimes, in which the same souls reincarnated together in different roles.

GROUP SUPPORT

Group meetings, bringing together people with the same medical condition, can enhance coping and relieve distress. Some of the clinical trials on cancer patient populations have reported that those who attend groups survive longer than those who do not, though other studies have not confirmed this. There are many different styles of group, ranging from self-help support run by patients themselves to educational or psychotherapeutic interventions led by professionals. On-line communities can serve a similar function and are more suitable for those who prefer anonymity or are unable to attend meetings.

The benefits of group support come from exchanging information about treatments and ways of coping, and from the empathic understanding which can only be provided by others 'in the same boat'. Even for those with caring family and friends, being ill can be an isolating experience: 'The feelings of being very alone, even while I have such wonderful love and support from so many, is unexpected'.

However not everyone wants to take part in group discussions and there are potential disadvantages, for example dealing with 'awkward' members, observing others deteriorate or die, and encouraging too much preoccupation with illness-related topics.

Besides providing benefits for their own members, support groups and patient organisations have a role in educating the wider community about medical conditions, and reducing the stigma which some of these carry. Public attitudes can change markedly over time; in the early days of my medical career, for example, the word 'cancer' aroused so much fear, and sometimes shame, that the diagnosis was often kept secret within families or even withheld from patients themselves. Now it is openly talked about, and attracts a great deal of interest, sympathy and funding, depending to some extent on the primary site; breast cancer has a better public profile than, say, cancer of the head and neck. Two other examples of conditions which are much less stigmatised than they used to be are AIDS and eating disorders. These changes can be attributed at least in part to patients speaking out about their disease, and campaigning for better treatment and support. Some conditions still tend to attract negative assumptions which may be unjustified, for example that skin disease always results from poor personal hygiene, sexually transmitted infection from promiscuity, or obesity from laziness and greed. Other conditions are stigmatised because they are poorly understood; one of these is migraine, which has overshadowed my own life for many years.

Unless they have experienced it themselves, few people seem to appreciate the intense suffering caused by a migraine attack or the lifestyle restrictions imposed by this disease, and many sufferers feel that they are dismissed as neurotics or malingerers.

ANIMAL COMPANIONSHIP

As an animal lover myself, I know how rewarding animal companionship can be. Many studies have confirmed the physical and mental health benefits of owning a pet, and the value of animal-assisted therapies such as riding for the disabled and having visiting dogs in hospices and care homes. Some of the benefits are mediated through increased exercise, but others are a direct result of the human-animal bond, which usually represents a form of pure unconditional love free from the complications which so often beset human relationships. Positive interaction with a dog, for example, leads to increased secretion of the 'love hormone' oxytocin, which has cardioprotective effects. Dog ownership is associated with a reduced risk of heart disease, and with a greatly improved prognosis for men who have had a heart attack already, although this may partly reflect the fact that men who choose to keep a dog are fitter to start off with.

The other side to this is that the death of a pet can be followed by a grief reaction similar to that which follows human bereavement, and in a few cases this can be just as severe, with adverse consequences for mental and physical health.

PROFESSIONAL RELATIONSHIPS

The next two sections are addressed to readers who are providing healthcare, whether in the orthodox or alternative field, rather than to those on the receiving end. However, the roles of 'healer' and 'healee' often overlap. Many of us will experience both these roles at different stages of life. Sometimes they run in parallel; many people in the healthcare professions are continuing to work while coping with chronic illness themselves, and many lay people with chronic illness are providing informal care to family members. Good doctors, nurses and other clinicians will readily admit that they are continually learning from their patients and clients. And patients who are assertive enough can sometimes offer the less good clinicians some tactful guidance.

The way that practitioners relate to their patients, or clients, can have a huge impact on the illness experience. Strong trusting relationships with healthcare professionals can do a great deal to relieve distress and promote recovery. An unhurried and empathetic first consultation, followed by a co-operative ongoing therapeutic partnership, is always helpful and in some contexts may contribute just as much to the healing process as the specific therapy given. A treatment given in a sympathetic and friendly atmosphere may feel entirely different from the same procedure delivered by staff who seem critical or uncaring.

The value of 'good communication skills' in medicine is widely recognised in theory, but unfortunately there still exists a minority of clinicians who are blunt, arrogant, patronising or even brutal in the way they talk and behave towards their patients. Perhaps they are under the illusion that all their theoretical knowledge and technical skill sets them up on a pedestal from which they are entitled to look down upon common humanity. Poor communication between doctors and patients is a factor in the majority of formal complaints processed by the General Medical Council in the UK.

Most orthodox clinicians, however, are genuinely concerned for their patients, and some of them would like to be able to practise in a more holistic way. They may have entered their professions with a strong sense of vocation, only to find this incompletely fulfilled in their highly specialised work environments where the emphasis on evidence-based and cost-effective methods tends to reduce scope for compassionate personalised medicine, as described in Robin Youngson's book *Time to care*. They wish to revive the 'art' of healthcare, the 'heart and soul' of their calling, and would be interested in exploring broader perspectives on healing but are constrained within the framework of the medical model. With much of orthodox practice now being carried out according to standard guidelines informed by the results of diagnostic tests, and with clinicians having to spend so much time in meetings or on computers, there is limited scope for detailed history-taking, clinical examination, discussion of diagnosis and treatment options, and getting to know each patient as an individual person.

Given these constraints, it is always possible to treat patients with courtesy and respect. The following points of guidance, addressed to healthcare practitioners, can help to establish good therapeutic relationships:

- Choosing words with care: Just as taking a drug can trigger a placebo or nocebo effect, so can hearing an authoritative statement from a healthcare practitioner,
- Providing adequate information: I know from personal experience that, even today, many clinicians in both the public and private sectors fail to put their patients fully in the picture regarding the results of investigations or the potential side-effects of treatments,
- Being honest: When there is 'bad news' about diagnosis and prognosis, telling the truth while still maintaining hope is a fine art. Being prepared to admit when you do not know all the answers, or have made a mistake, will usually increase rather than decrease patients' respect,
- Listening: Allowing patients to say what is important to them and attending with understanding and interest, rather than making judgements or assumptions or trying to fix the problem with unasked-for advice,
- Learning something about patients' personal and social life: Besides helping to establish good working relationships, this can elicit information which is relevant to future management. An unduly narrow approach might miss, for example, that someone is unable to

comply properly with treatment because they are caring for a disabled spouse; has a past history of psychosis and may need assessment by the mental health team during their surgical admission; cannot follow an instruction leaflet because of inability to read and write; or knows more about the illness in question than the clinician does,
- Self-disclosure: Within limits, this can be helpful. If you or someone in your family has suffered from the same condition as your patient, consider sharing some of this experience, without letting the consultation become focused on your own troubles. Providing your private phone number in case of emergencies is reassuring for patients and occasionally very useful, and hardly any of them will abuse the privilege,
- Kindness: Kind words from a clinician can have a powerful healing effect. And, however senior your professional position, be aware of opportunities to carry out a simple act of kindness such as moving a patient's meal tray within reach.

SELF-CARE FOR HEALERS

The following guidelines, like those in the previous section, are addressed directly to professional clinicians. Many of them are also relevant to voluntary care-givers, such as people looking after a sick family member, and indeed to anyone whose work involves some kind of service to others.

Healthcare practitioners do not always enjoy good health themselves, perhaps because of the stressful nature of their work, and a tendency to neglect their own self-care because they consider themselves immune from the ailments which afflict their patients. Mental health problems such as 'burnout', alcohol and drug abuse, and suicide are particular risks in the medical profession. Nobody can do their best work if their own condition is under par.

The following guidelines may help to prevent problems.

- Setting boundaries against excessive work demands: This ensures time to eat regular meals, get enough sleep, take some outdoor exercise, maintain relationships with family and friends, and pursue interests outside medicine,
- Maintaining emotional outlets: Such as talking to confidants, and expressive activities such as writing, music, sport or dance,
- Aiming for the right balance between caring so deeply for your patients that you take on their problems and become emotionally exhausted, and becoming so detached or cynical that you lose empathy and compassion,
- Keeping values in mind: If much of your time and energy is being spent studying for higher qualifications, negotiating with managers, coping with awkward colleagues or simply getting through a heavy workload in time to get home at a reasonable hour, it is easy to forget that you went into your profession to help sick people.

Those whose job it is to heal others sometimes expect to always be in perfect health themselves, regarding personal illness as a sign of weakness or incompetence. In fact, even with the best of self-care, nearly everyone gets sick sometimes and the human body has a limited life span. 'Wounded healers' who have experienced and learned from their own experience of sickness can be the most powerful healers of all.

PART 6

External Treatments

Decisions about the management of illness can depend on individual preferences and priorities. Whether to seek professional treatments or rely on self-help techniques? Whether to take the orthodox or the alternative path? Whether to undertake a gruelling treatment in the hope of improving long-term prognosis, or to focus on optimising quality of life in the present? Whether the best interests of patient or family come first, in cases where they are not aligned? Though it is sometimes necessary to make a choice between two options which are not compatible with each other, it is often possible to find a satisfactory compromise.

PROFESSIONAL TREATMENTS OR SELF-HELP?

When there is serious threat to life or health it is clearly essential to seek expert treatment and care. Less serious conditions often recover on their own, or can be successfully managed with self-help measures, but there are still advantages in having a professional assessment from someone who can view the situation from a different perspective and explain the results of clinical examination and diagnostic tests, so making it easier to reach informed decisions about management. Early diagnosis and treatment of some diseases offers an improved chance of cure. Even in cases of terminal illness, both orthodox and CAM treatments can help with relieving physical symptoms and improving psychological and spiritual adjustment.

The challenge lies in finding a balance between benefiting from professional expertise, and retaining personal responsibility for health. In developed countries in recent years there has been a tendency for people to hand over too much control of their bodies and minds to healthcare professionals, due to a growing 'medicalisation' of everyday life. The professionals involved are usually acting with the best of intentions, and may not have considered that investigating and treating more people means higher incomes and enhanced career prospects for orthodox clinicians, natural therapists, employees of drug companies, and suppliers of natural remedies.

A broadening of the diagnostic criteria for existing diseases, and the discovery or concoction of new ones, has meant that people going through a normal stage of development, or experiencing appropriate variations in emotions and behaviour, are now more likely to be labelled as having a physical or mental disorder. Also, the introduction of general population screening programmes has led to large numbers being started on treatment for 'borderline abnormalities' or 'risk factors' discovered on routine examinations or blood tests. At the time of writing it is being proposed that everyone in the UK over the age of 50 should start taking a daily 'polypill' to reduce the risk of cardiovascular disease. If this happens, time will tell whether the anticipated benefits for the majority will outweigh the drug-induced problems which some users will undoubtedly develop, but history shows that such mass medication can have unfortunate results. Not so long ago, for example, women were being encouraged to remain 'feminine forever' by taking hormone replacement therapy (HRT) after menopause, but this advice was changed after clinical trials identified an increased risk of breast cancer, heart disease and stroke attributable to these drugs. HRT does carry some benefits, such as helping to prevent osteoporosis, but is now only recommended when there are strong clinical indications in the individual case.

The wisdom of starting long-term preventive medications or carrying out surgical procedures for symptom-free people on the basis of medical tests can often be questioned. There is, for example, current controversy about the value of prescribing drugs for mild hypertension, and of treating early cases of breast or prostate cancer which have been detected by screening. For some of those concerned, prompt treatment will indeed save life and health, because their condition would have progressed without it. Unfortunately there is no reliable way of telling these people apart from the many others who will be wrongly diagnosed as having a disease, burdened with groundless anxiety, and harmed by the unwanted effects of unnecessary drugs or surgery.

There are no easy answers to such dilemmas but it is likely that many of those who are found to have borderline abnormalities or risk factors, as opposed to clinically evident disease, could be managed by lifestyle adjustment along with continued observation. The health benefits of safe natural measures such as having enough exercise, sleep and relaxation, eating plenty of fresh vegetables and fruit, moderate exposure to sunlight, strong personal relationships, stress reduction and a positive mental outlook have long been emphasised in holistic healing circles, and are now well documented in the orthodox literature too. In recent years such measures have received more attention in orthodox medicine, and are emphasised in public health education programmes aimed at preventing disease. The efficacy and safety of certain traditional home remedies, ginger for the treatment of nausea for example, have also been confirmed in formal studies. However such simple things are often ignored in medical settings, where patients are commonly prescribed drugs or surgery without being advised about their diet or way of life.

ORTHODOX OR ALTERNATIVE?

As already stated, both mainstream treatments and natural therapies can form part of a holistic programme, and it is often better to think in terms of 'complementary' or 'integrative' medicine instead of drawing a rigid dividing line between the 'orthodox' and 'alternative'. However, there is still a tendency to regard these two approaches as polar opposites which are incompatible with each other or even at war.

Both among clinicians and patients, attitudes vary enormously. Some orthodox doctors and nurses have an active interest in the holistic approach, and may have undertaken training in a CAM modality such as acupuncture or homoeopathy themselves. Some, though they might be sympathetic in theory, learned little or nothing about such topics during their training and when patients ask about them they do not have either the time or the knowledge to give an effective response. A few are frankly hostile, and controversy tends to rage especially high in cancer care settings. Examples of dismissive or negative statements made by oncologists, as reported to me by their patients, include 'I'm afraid there's absolutely nothing you can do except have the radiotherapy', 'I don't mind if you want to try that but you know perfectly well it won't make any difference' and even 'I will refuse to continue treating you if you go in for anything like that'. Rather than risk such responses, many patients who are using or considering CAM conceal the fact from their doctors. Media reports relating to well-known people such as John Diamond, Steve Jobs, Christopher Hitchens and Iain Banks who have died from cancer in recent years often include strongly-worded opinions either for or against the use of anything alternative.

There are several reasons for negative attitudes to CAM, some more valid than others. Advocates of evidence-based medicine may consider the research foundation inadequate. Opponents may be defensively over-reacting to a perceived threat of challenge to their authority coming from an alien source which they do not understand. They may be over-generalising from a single case in which a therapy was misused with tragic results, or from an encounter with an alternative therapist who was incompetent, fraudulent or deluded. Or they may fear medico-legal reprisals if they seem to be departing from standard treatment protocols or endorsing unproven treatments.

Some tenets of the holistic approach, the importance of good nutrition and of good therapeutic relationships for example, are already widely accepted in orthodox circles at least in principle. Others, involving for example 'subtle energies' and spiritual forces, are more esoteric and often quite unfamiliar to those with an orthodox training and scepticism about such concepts is another of the reasons which make some orthodox clinicians determined to attack and destroy the practice of CAM. Homoeopathy has been the target of especially virulent criticism although it is used by millions of people worldwide, in some countries being the main system of healthcare, and although its efficacy is supported by many research studies. Critics assume that homoeopathy cannot possibly work because its mode of action is not explained by the orthodox scientific paradigm. It was denounced as 'witchcraft' at a conference of the British Medical Association in 2010, and in 2013 the UK's Chief Medical Officer called it 'rubbish'.

On the other side of the coin, a few CAM practitioners are totally opposed to orthodox medicine, for example condemning all pharmaceutical drugs as evil poisons. This can create dilemmas for patients who are seeking complementary support alongside orthodox treatment, for example the woman with breast cancer who did not know what to do when her oncologist recommended chemotherapy but her naturopath told her not to have it. Some patients are themselves determined to avoid conventional treatments at all costs; I know of one man, a passionate advocate of alternative medicine, who died at a relatively young age from an overwhelming infection after he had absolutely refused on principle to accept the antibiotic treatment which would probably have saved his life. I know others who spent large amounts of time and money on natural therapies without benefit, and then reluctantly accepted conventional treatment which brought about complete recovery.

There are some points on which allopathic and alternative practitioners will never agree. For example, most orthodox public health experts recommend immunisation and vaccination programmes for the population at large, whereas most homoeopaths are very much against these interventions. On the majority of issues, however, there is plenty of scope for agreement and compromise, and it would be helpful for patients if there were more communication and co-operation between the two professional camps.

Having decided to accept external treatment of whatever kind, it is a good idea to undertake it with a whole-hearted commitment. People who have hope and faith that it is going to work are more likely to benefit than those who have reluctantly agreed to have it in a spirit of resentment and doubt. At the same time it is important to be aware that almost all external treatments, whether mainstream or CAM, carry some degree of risk.

CAUTIONS WITH DRUGS AND SURGERY

Modern medicine and surgery can achieve wonderful results when appropriately used. They often make the difference between life and death for patients with acute disorders such as heart attack, diabetic coma, overwhelming infections, bowel obstruction or traumatic injury; restore quality of life for those with chronic disorders such as arthritis of the hip or cataracts of the eye; and relieve the symptoms of those dying from incurable disease. The following paragraphs, however, are concerned with the potential downside of orthodox treatments in cases where they are not essential and their value may not be established.

Many authorities would agree that pharmaceutical medications are over-prescribed today, and that there are many good reasons for curbing their use. They are, in the main, much more powerful than 'natural' remedies and as such they carry great potential to cause harm as well as good. Prescribed drugs, whether taken as directed or as the means of overdose, now cause more deaths than road traffic accidents in the United States.

All pharmaceuticals can have unwanted effects, which need to be balanced against their benefits. For example the regular use of anti-inflammatory drugs such as ibuprofen increases the risks of heart attack, stroke and bleeding from the gut, though many patients are willing to accept these risks as the price to pay for controlling symptoms such as the pain of arthritis. When and if more drugs are added to counteract unwanted effects of the first prescription, the ingredients of this chemical cocktail can interact to cause new symptoms which can be impossible to disentangle from those of the original disorder.

Other points of concern include the rise of untreatable bacterial infections which has followed the over-prescribing of antibiotics; the risks of dependence and abuse with some psychotropics and analgesics; the suffering of the animals on which new drugs have to be tested in the course of development; pollution of the water supply by excreted or discarded pharmaceuticals; the dubious nature of certain marketing tactics employed by 'Big Pharma' (Healy 2012); and the financial costs of medication.

As regards surgery, operations which are carried out for good reasons by skilled surgeons usually have successful results and sometimes the outcome is excellent. However all operations carry some risk, whether associated with the anaesthetic or with the procedure itself. Whereas the unwanted effects of medication usually recover when the drug is stopped, those resulting from surgery are quite often permanent, and attempts to improve the situation with further surgery do not always work and may even make things worse. A consultant in a teaching hospital, demonstrating the case of a very sick woman to his medical students, said 'This patient has had five abdominal operations - and only the first one was not necessary.' Before going ahead with a non-essential operation such as hysterectomy for fibroids, cholecystectomy for gallstones, or any kind of preventive or cosmetic procedure, it is wise to weigh up the likely benefits and risks with great care.

A criticism which is sometimes directed towards orthodox treatments is that they merely 'attack the disease' or 'suppress the symptoms', whereas natural therapies such as homoeopathy are claimed to correct the 'root causes' of ill-health and stimulate the body's own defences. This is an over-generalisation but does contain some truth. One example would be 'waging the war on cancer' with the conventional 'cut, poison and burn' approach, rather than pursuing therapies designed to prevent or cure this disease by avoiding risk factors and strengthening the immune system. Other examples involve the use of antibiotics, steroids or analgesics for minor conditions, which may be rapidly effective in controlling the symptoms but according to their critics can drive the pathology deeper into the body leading to more serious illness later on.

Clearly, it is humane to try to relieve symptoms which are causing significant distress, but it is also worth considering that these symptoms may be serving a purpose as the body's way of trying to correct an imbalance, in other words to restore homeostasis. Examples of this would be the elimination of toxins through vomiting, diarrhoea, sweating or skin eruptions. The relief of suffering should not be used as a substitute for attempting to address its cause. My colleague Jasmine Sampson (www.How-to-create-miracles.com) gives the example of a high-achieving woman who worked very long hours, including weekends, in her business. She began to suffer from migraines and visited her doctor who recommended she cut back her hours and gave her some pain relief tablets. Rather than cutting back her hours, she used the tablets to control the pain so she could carry on as before. A little while later she suffered a stroke and had to stop work altogether.

CAUTIONS WITH CAM

In view of the potential risks of orthodox medicine and surgery as summarised above, it may seem tempting to stick to natural approaches. CAM therapies tend to be gentler than allopathic treatments, and are less likely to cause major damage. However 'natural' is not equivalent to 'safe' and some natural treatments can be harmful. For example, acupuncture needles can cause injury or infection if improperly applied. Herbal remedies and nutritional supplements can have unwanted effects, especially if they contain toxic impurities.

Most natural therapies can safely be used alongside orthodox treatments but there are some herbal medicines and dietary supplements which are known to interact with certain pharmaceutical drugs, either rendering them less effective, or increasing the risk of unwanted effects. There are probably many more potential interactions which have not been recognised. It is therefore advisable for patients to tell their doctors if they are using CAM, although many in fact do not.

The relative lack of regulation governing the CAM field means that there is little safeguard against useless or harmful therapies, and against fraudulent or incompetent practitioners.

Even when natural therapies are being used correctly, they can sometimes cause people to feel worse before they feel better due to the so-called 'healing reactions' which develop in a minority of cases. There may be an aggravation of the current symptoms; or the return of old symptoms from the past; or 'cleansing' phenomena such as skin rashes or diarrhoea. This indicates that the chosen therapy is resonating with the person and so will probably have beneficial results in the longer term. Healing reactions are usually mild and temporary, but sensitive subjects may find them distressing especially if they had not been warned that they might occur. In the event of a marked healing reaction it is best to contact a qualified therapist, who may recommend modifying the treatment regime. It is important to bear in mind that the symptoms may not be due to a healing reaction at all, but to something different such as an allergy or infection which requires treatment in its own right.

An indirect danger is that of using alternative approaches, as opposed to complementary ones, in situations where orthodox medicine or surgery would have been more effective. CAM therapies, being less powerful than allopathic treatments, seldom provide adequate treatment for a serious disease when used on their own. Prosecutions have been directed at parents whose children have died after being given unproven therapies for cancers which could probably have been cured by conventional treatment.

In many ways, allopathic and natural treatments are truly complementary to each other. Integrative medicine, designed to combine and co-ordinate elements of both approaches as tailored to the individual case, could be the best way forward for the future but at present is only available from a few experts in a few centres. People on the 'illness journey' who choose to depart from the main highway of orthodox treatment sometimes find themselves on a rather lonely path without clear maps or easy access to support services.

CONSIDERING THE AIMS OF TREATMENT

Cure or control of the disease process itself, and relief of its physical or mental symptoms, often go hand in hand but they are not the same thing. Sometimes both can be covered by the same treatment, but sometimes they require different approaches, as in the case of the woman described above who used drugs to mask her migraine symptoms without addressing the imbalance in her lifestyle.

Good physical self-care and a positive mental attitude tend to be associated with improvements in immune function, hormone profile and other physiological measures. For people with serious disease, therefore, quality of life and length of life tend to go together rather than being mutually exclusive. In other words, living better often means living longer. A controlled study of patients with lung cancer showed that those given an early referral to palliative care services, which incorporate many of the principles of the holistic approach, lived longer than those receiving routine care (Ternel et al 2010). Some randomised trials involving patients with various forms of cancer have shown a survival advantage for those receiving effective psychological support (Spiegel 2012), though other studies have not confirmed this.

There are some situations which do call for making a choice between the best possible quality of life and the best possible medical prognosis. The decisions involved can be very difficult, and the balance between the different options may change over time. The woman described earlier, diagnosed with a cancer of the mouth which had spread to the lymph nodes in her neck, was advised to undergo extensive surgery followed by radiotherapy and chemotherapy. This radical course of treatment offered only a limited hope of cure and would carry many unwanted effects including the need to have all her teeth removed, which horrified her. Without the treatment, she was advised that she would 'die a horrible death within 12 months'. She wrote at that time 'I read the booklets all about radiation and chemo. The damage caused is so against what I have always believed, that you don't poison the world or the body you live in, that I would not be living my own truth to go that way. I thought about the time they said I would have left if I didn't do their treatment and decided I could live with that and would do the best I knew how and enjoy it. I have stopped work and now do what I feel is good and right for us all.' As well as making the courageous decisions to decline orthodox treatments and to resolve her unhappy living circumstances, she used homoeopathic and herbal remedies and many other natural treatments from reputable alternative practitioners, with the loving support of her new partner and her family. Despite all this the cancer continued to grow, making it hard to talk or swallow, and in her last email to me she wrote of having to 'bite the bullet' of accepting radiotherapy. But within a few weeks she died, and to quote from her death notice she 'passed away after being diagnosed with cancer and bravely focusing on quality of life, getting the best out of each day and doing it her way'.

CHOOSING COMPLEMENTARY THERAPIES

People often ask how they can choose among the hundreds of CAM therapies available. There is no easy answer to this question because there have been few studies making direct comparisons between different therapies for the same condition. In any case the value of such comparisons would be limited in the light of the axiom 'treat the patient not the disease'. Having said this, there are plenty of research studies about individual CAM therapies in the literature, which can be searched through websites such as nccam.nih.gov and www.rccm.org.uk.

Most CAM interventions are intended to stimulate the self-healing response as it involves the whole person. This is in contrast to most pharmaceutical drugs, which are designed to target a single chemical process with the minimum of generalised effects. While it would be going too far to regard all natural therapies as interchangeable, there is considerable scope for overlap between them, and a single 'best' therapy for the disorder in question may not exist. Some of the benefits are specific to particular interventions but other factors such as the relationship with the therapist, belief in the value of the therapy, and the practicalities of obtaining it locally are important to take into account. Sometimes an apparently random choice can be successful, as in the following case:

'Ten years ago, while working in the secretarial and administrative section of a large office, I developed pain in both elbows. The pain grew to become heat, swelling and stiffness. It was some months later that I realised my physical symptoms had started within two weeks of a change in word processing packages, involving hot keys, key usage and adjusting body position to the new keyboards and screens.

'The unwellness spread quickly upwards, from both elbows to both shoulders. After that the achy pain, sore muscles, throbbing, heat and swelling crept slowly back downwards into my fingers and knuckles. My hands were sore, hard, swollen and with little dexterity or flexibility. For months on end I was in a lot of pain, not only during the day, but much worse at night. The only way to sleep was with my arms upright in the air! Eventually I was unable to type, unable to carry anything with my arms and fingers and felt as though I had become partly crippled. This occurred over a year-long period.

'A friend recommended I see a Classical Homoeopath, which I did promptly. Might I add I had absolutely no idea of what 'that' meant. I attended several sessions, and made several follow up phone calls to the Homoeopath over several months which entailed taking and repeating a homoeopathic remedy under precise instructions.

'Initially it felt as though my condition had worsened. A month later my hands were much more painful but my shoulders were improving. Over the next two months, so all in all three months after treatment began, I was almost better, just a few niggly pains in my knuckles, which later disappeared as well.

'I have to admit to being sceptical of the treatment – except for the fact that numerous visits to the orthodox doctor had ended in no satisfaction or intuitive feeling of cure being even mildly possible. I had been diagnosed with RSI – repetitive strain injury.

'I enjoyed the Homoeopathic consultations, but found the questions often difficult to answer. Yet over time, the questions began to open my mind to my own healing process.

'I had a mild relapse many years later – I mean 'mild', only slightly achy in the elbows and fingers. This was easily cured and life meanwhile for me returned to absolute normal.'

This woman went on to train as a homoeopath herself, developing a thriving practice and, like most other homoeopaths I have known, passionate about her work.

No single type of treatment works for everyone, so it may be necessary to try several natural therapies before finding what helps, while at the same time giving each one a fair chance. The benefits of CAM usually build up gradually, sometimes over months rather than weeks, and some people feel worse before they feel better due to the development of 'healing reactions' as described above. Therefore it is often a mistake to give up after just a few days of using a self-help technique or having just a single session with a therapist.

It is quite common practice to use two or more natural therapies together, combining those which work primarily at the physical level with other approaches of a more psychological or spiritual kind, and with self-help techniques. This may seem rather 'unscientific' because it makes it impossible to tell which is having an effect and because certain therapies either overlap or clash with each other, but often no single intervention is enough on its own.

During 40 years of living with migraines I tried many prescribed drugs, natural therapies and special diets in turn, searching for 'the' remedy which would prevent or treat the horrible attacks of headache, nausea and vomiting. I embarked on each new approach with high hopes, which were always dashed before long. Contrary to expectation the episodes became worse and more frequent following menopause, even though I had retired from full-time work and was leading a happy life without any obvious stress. Then more recently, since I gave up searching for a 'magic bullet' and just aimed to follow a healthy lifestyle incorporating some of the self-help techniques described above, they have become much less frequent and less severe. Perhaps I am 'growing out' of migraine at last, as sometimes happens in later life; perhaps all the various things I am doing to support my health are working; perhaps I have taken on board the 'lessons' the condition was trying to teach me. Without it, I certainly doubt whether I would have explored all the various paths to healing which I write about in my books.

There is a widespread expectation that health will worsen with increasing age, and although this does of course prove true for some people, for others the opposite happens. I have several friends who were diagnosed with advanced heart disease or other serious conditions in their 40s or 50s, and prepared themselves for an early death, but now in their 60s or 70s are living healthy active lives. None of them attribute their improvement to a single factor, but they have all used some combination of medical treatments and complementary therapies, have retired from demanding jobs or resolved discord in relationships, and are spending time on things they enjoy.

It is never too late to give up in the face of a long-standing illness. Through combining the best of both orthodox and natural medicine with self-care of the body, mind and spirit there is always hope of kindling the healing response.

APPENDIX

Alphabetical list of complementary therapies

This is by no means a complete list of the many approaches available, but includes a selection of widely-used modalities. Some of them can be used on a self-help basis but are most are better undertaken with the guidance of a qualified therapist.

I have not included references with this list because there are so many different books, websites and research papers available that in most cases it is not possible to recommend a single definitive source. Searching on Google by the name of the therapy combined with the name of the symptom or disease in question (examples: 'homoeopathy and headache' or 'reflexology and arthritis') will probably yield thousands of results and it is important to look at several of the different websites listed because their quality will be variable, some being commercially driven rather than clinically sound. Searching on www.ncbi.nim.nih.gov/pubmed will produce a much smaller number of results limited to academic publications from the biomedical literature. If little or nothing is found there it does not necessarily mean that the therapy is ineffective for the condition in question, just that no relevant studies have been done. Remember that, being focused on 'persons not diseases', most of the therapies are designed to bring the whole system into balance rather than treating a particular symptom in isolation.

Another way of finding information is to search the internet for the training schools and professional societies for particular therapies in your country of residence. Their websites often provide information about what is involved, and lists of qualified practitioners.

Acupuncture
Anthroposophy
Aromatherapy
Art therapy
Ayurveda
Bach flower remedies
Bodytalk
Chiropractic
Colour therapy
Emotional freedom technique (EFT, tapping)
Herbal medicine
Homoeopathy (also spelled homeopathy)
Hypnotherapy
Kinesiology
Massage
Music therapy
Naturopathy
Neurolinguistic programming (NLP)
Nutritional therapy
Osteopathy
PsychK
Quantum touch
Reflexology
Reiki
Spiritual healing
Therapeutic touch
Traditional Chinese Medicine
Yoga

REFERENCES

Bach, E. (1931). Heal thyself. Available as a free download from www.bachcentre.com/centre/download/heal_thy.pdf.

Benor, D.J. (2007). Spiritual healing: scientific validation of a healing revolution. Wholistic Healing Publications.

Benson, H., Dusek J.A., Sherwood J.B. et al (2006). Study of the therapeutic effects of intercessionary prayer (STEP) in cardiac bypass patients. American Heart Journal 151 (4) 934-42.

Benson, H. and Proctor, W. (2011). Relaxation Revolution: the science and genetics of mind body healing. Scribner.

Bishop, B. (2005). A time to heal. First Stone.

Bosma H., Marmot M.G., Hemingway H. et al (1997). Low job control and risk of coronary heart disease in whitehall ii (prospective cohort) study. British Medical Journal 314 558-65.

Bunker, S.J., Colquhoun, D.M, Esler, M.D. et al (2003). 'Stress' and coronary heart disease: psychosocial risk factors. Medical Journal of Australia 178 (6) 272-276.

Chida, Y. and Steptoe, A. (2008). Positive psychological well-being and mortality: a quantitative review of prospective observational studies. Psychosomatic Medicine 70 (7) 741-56.

Doidge, N. (2007). The brain that changes itself: stories of personal triumph from the frontiers of brain science. Viking.

Dossey, L. (1993). Healing words: the power of prayer and the practice of medicine. HarperSanFrancisco.

Dossey, L. (1999). Reinventing medicine. HarperSanFrancisco.

Essex, A. (2013). Practical miracles: choices that heal and build resilience. Hay House.

Estruch, R., Ros, E., Salas-Salvado, J. et al (2013). Primary prevention of cardiovascular disease with a Mediterranean diet. New England Journal of Medicine 368 1279-90.

Fang, F., Fall, K., Mittleman, M.A. et al (2012). Suicide and cardiovascular death after a cancer diagnosis. New England Journal of Medicine 366 1310-18.

Gawain, S. (2002). Creative visualisation: use the power of your imagination to create what you want in your life. New World Library.

Gawler, I. (2012). You can conquer cancer. Michelle Anderson.

Gerber, R. (2000). A practical guide to vibrational medicine: energy healing and spiritual transformation. Harper Collins.

Giltay, E.J., Geleijnse J.M., Zitman F.G. et al (2004). Dispositional optimism and all-cause and cardiovascular mortality in a prospective cohort of elderly Dutch men and women. Archives of General Psychiatry 61 (11) 1126-35.

Gramling, R., Klein, W., Roberts, M. et al (2008). Self-rated cardiovascular risk and 15-year cardiovascular mortality. Annals of Family Medicine 6 (4) 302-6.

Green, A.R., Carrillo, J.E., Betancourt, J.R. (2002). Why the disease-based model of medicine fails our patients. Western Journal of Medicine 176 (2) 141-3.

Hamilton, D. (2008). How your mind can heal your body. Hay House.

Harris, P.E., Cooper, K.L., Relton, C., Thomas, K.J. (2012). Prevalence of complementary and alternative medicine (CAM) use by the general population: a systematic review and update. International Journal of Clinical Practice 66(10) 924-39.

Hay, L. (1984). You can heal your life. Hay House.

Healy, D. (2012). Pharmageddon. University of California Press.

Hirshberg, C. and Barasch, M. (1995). Remarkable recovery: what extraordinary healings tell us about getting well and staying well. Riverhead Books.

Kelly, R. (2011). The human hologram. Energy Psychology Press.

Lang, F.R., Weiss, D., Gerstoff, D., Wagner, G.G. (2013). Forecasting life satisfaction across adulthood: benefits of seeing a dark future? Psychology and Aging 28 (1) 249-61.

LeShan, L. (1994). Cancer as a turning point: a handbook for people with cancer, their families, and health professionals. Plume Penguin.

Levenstein S. (1998). Stress and peptic ulcer: life beyond helicobacter. British Medical Journal 316 538-41.

Lipton, B. (2008). The biology of belief: unleashing the power of consciousness, matter and miracles. Hay House.

Ludwig, D.S., Kabat-Zinn, J. (2008). Mindfulness in medicine. Journal of the American Medical Association 300 (11) 1350-1352.

Moorjani, A. (2012). Dying to be me: my journey from cancer, to near death, to true healing. Hay House.

Ober, C., Sinatra, S.T. and Zucker, M.(2010). Earthing: the most important health discovery ever? Basic Health Publications.

Rankin, L. (2013). Mind over medicine: scientific proof that you can heal yourself. Hay House.

Rendall, M.S., Weden, M.M., Favreault, M.M., Waldron, H. (2011). The protective effect of marriage for survival: a review and update. Demography 48(2) 481-506.

Russ, T.C., Stamatakis, E., Hamer, M. et al (2012). Association between psychological distress and mortality: individual participant pooled analysis of 10 prospective cohort studies. British Medical Journal 345; e4933.

Siegel, B. (1998). Love, medicine and miracles: lessons learned about self-healing from a surgeon's experience with exceptional patients. Harper Collins.

Simonton, C.O., Matthews-Simonton, S., Creighton, J.L. (1992). Getting Well Again. Bantam Books.

Spiegel, D. (2012). Mind matters in cancer survival. Psychooncology 21 (6) 588-93.

Ternel, J.S., Greer, J.A., Muzikansky, A., et al. (2010). Early palliative care for patients with metastatic non-small-cell lung cancer. New England Journal of Medicine 363 (8) 733-42.

Uchino, B.N. (2006). Social support and health: a review of physiological processes potentially underlying links to disease outcomes. Journal of Behavioural Medicine 29 (4) 377-87.

Ulrich, R.S. (1984). View through a window may influence recovery from surgery. Science 224 420-21.

Ware, B. (2012). The five top regrets of the dying: a life transformed by the dearly departing. Hay House.

Youngson, R. (2012). Time to care: how to love your patients and your job. Rebelheart.

ABOUT THE AUTHOR

Jennifer Barraclough lives with her husband and cats in Auckland, New Zealand. She originally comes from England, where she worked as a medical doctor before retraining as a Bach flower practitioner and life coach. She has written or edited eight previous books including *Enhancing cancer care: complementary therapy and support*; *Focus on healing: holistic self-help for medical illness*; *Life's labyrinth; the path and the purpose*; and *Bach flowers for mind-body healing*.

Printed in Great Britain
by Amazon